# Drop a
# Dress Size

This is a Parragon book
This edition published in 2005

Parragon
Queen Street House
4 Queen Street
Bath, BA1 1HE, UK

Contributing Editor
Maggie Pannell

This edition designed by
Design Principals, Warminster

ISBN 1-40544-795-8
Printed in China

**DISCLAIMER**

The exercises and advice detailed in this book assume that you are a normally healthy adult. Therefore the author, publishers, their servants, or agents cannot accept responsibility for loss or damage suffered by individuals as a result of following advice or attempting an exercise or treatment referred to in this book. It is strongly recommended that individuals intending to undertake an exercise programme and any change of diet do so following consultation with their medical practitioner.

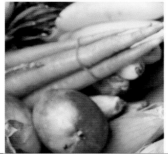

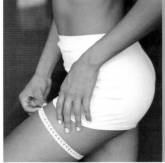

# Drop a Dress Size

an easy to follow

slimming and fitness plan

guaranteed to shift

inches as well as pounds

*p*

# Congratulations

Remember, weight loss is not the same as size loss, so exercises that concentrate on the parts of the body that affect your dress size the most, ie the bust, waist, tummy, hips and bottom, and fat burning activities like brisk walking, will shape and contour those vital statistics.

## Keep it up

Now that you have come this far, you don't want to risk slipping back into bad habits so the weight piles back on again and the dreaded cellulite returns. Keep up the changes you have made to your daily life by eating healthily and leading an active lifestyle. Once you're reached your target weight and size, you can increase the amount you eat, but stick to healthy eating guidelines (see pages 35-7, 47, 48). Remember the more active you are, the more you can eat as you'll be burning off those calories with the increased amount of energy used up.

## A new you!

Remove those over-sized garments that you had been wearing and were not happy with, from the wardrobe. You don't want them to be left hanging there as an easy option to slip back into. In fact, why not use this golden opportunity, to give your wardrobe a complete make-over. Ask a friend to help, not only to make the exercise more enjoyable but to also have a second and honest opinion as to what suits you and what doesn't. Clear out all the reject items and only retain the ones you like and feel good in. Above all, be proud of the way you look, enjoy your new shape and you can remain your perfect size forever.

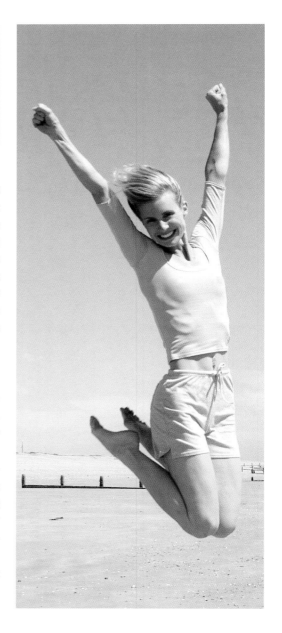

# Contents

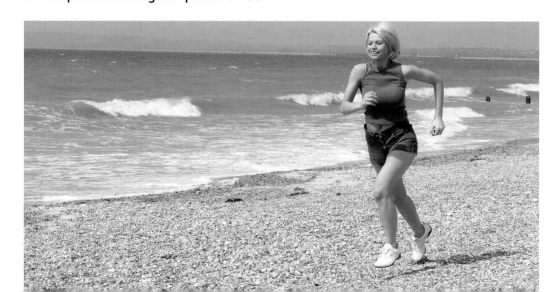

# Congratulations

It might not have been plain sailing, you may well have faltered along the way and succumbed to the occasional bar of chocolate, but that doesn't matter provided you've generally stuck with the healthy eating and regular exercise programme. And now your hard work, commitment and dedication are rewarded with the new size and shape you wanted. You will also feel healthier and more energized than you have done for ages. You can now look forward to the fun bit – shopping with confidence for those outfits you know you're going to look great in and wearing again those old favourites, previously relegated to the back of the wardrobe!

## Individual targets

Don't worry if you still have a little way to go to achieve that sylph-like figure you have long dreamed of. Remember everyone's metabolism is different and the time span it will take depends on how much weight you need to lose. You may have a fair amount of weight to lose to drop several dress sizes, in which case, although you will notice a significant weekly weight loss (1.8 –2.7 kg / 4-6 lb), you will need to follow the diet and exercise programme for longer to reach your goal. It is perfectly safe to continue for as long as you want to.

On the other hand, you may not have a lot of weight to lose but your uncomfortable measurements are due more to poor body tone or bad posture. If this is you, the scales may register only a small but steady weekly weight loss (1 – 1.4 kg / 2-3 lb) but following a regular exercise programme will produce the trimmer, firmer shape you are looking for in just 2-3 weeks. Don't become obsessive about your weight and frequently jump on the scales. A weekly weigh-in is all you need for a progress check. More importantly, if you've been following the workout routine, look in the mirror from time to time and you will soon notice improvements as your muscles become toned and strengthened.

**IN ORDER TO MAINTAIN YOUR NEW LOOK:**

- Continue eating 3 meals a day, although you can eat more than you did while slimming.
- Eat a wide variety of foods.
- Choose healthy snacks if you feel peckish between meals.
- Continue taking regular aerobic exercise, such as walking, cycling or swimming, as well as gradually building more activity into your daily life.
- Try to also continue with some muscle-toning exercises.
- Remember that good posture is important to how you look.
- Don't become obsessive about your weight. Weight fluctuates so don't keep hopping on and off the scales.
- Be proud of yourself and enjoy your new shape.

# Exercise plan

Dress size is a good indicator of your general health and fitness but to drop down to the size you want to be, it's not just a matter of eating healthily and losing a bit of weight. To get those curves in all the right places and to feel comfortable and sexy in your clothes, you also need to build regular exercise into your daily lifestyle.

When we are fit and active it can be much easier to find the motivation to let go of bad habits, such as smoking. So if you do smoke, now's a good time to try and give it up.

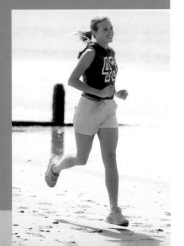

Active living will not only reward you with an enviable shape but will provide all kinds of other benefits associated with getting physical.

## The benefits of exercise

- improved feeling of well-being
- increased strength and flexibility
- more stamina
- reduced stress levels
- lowered blood pressure
- reduced cholesterol levels and a healthier heart
- weight loss
- better quality of sleep and alleviation of insomnia
- slowing down of the ageing process
- lower risk of late-onset diabetes
- relief of aches and pains
- increased levels of energy
- enhanced ability to recover from illness or injury
- better posture
- improved muscle tone
- improved health

## Why get fit?

There are many reasons for us to get fit and stay active and one of the main arguments is, possibly, because that is what we were designed to do. Man is an animal and until very recently in his history, his entire existence was centred around some kind of physical effort. Indeed, his very survival depended on it – his ability to be active allowed him to catch food, run away from his enemies, climb trees and cross rivers. Nowadays, with our reliance on technology and mechanisation, we no longer need to be physically active to survive in the outside world, yet our essential needs have not changed and in order to function effectively and efficiently our entire system – physical, mental and spiritual – requires daily activity. Also, it is not only our muscles that benefit from movement: our organs, glands and systems (circulation, digestion, respiration) become much more efficient when we are fit and active.

| FOOD | NUTRIENTS | BENEFITS | SERVING IDEAS |
|---|---|---|---|
| Chilli | • Vitamin C<br>• Beta-carotene<br>• Vitamin E<br>• Folate | • Stimulates circulation and helps prevent blood clots<br>• Eases coughs and colds, clearing congestion<br>• May protect the stomach against alcohol and acidic food<br>• Anticoagulant – helps to reduce blood pressure and cholesterol levels<br>• Stimulates the release of endorphins, the body's 'feel-good' chemicals | Use to spice up curries, stir-fries and marinades and for all kinds of exotic dishes. |
| Green Tea | • Quercetin (an antioxidant) | • The polyphenols in green tea help to protect against heart disease by reducing cholesterol levels, blood pressure and risk of blood clots<br>• May protect against some forms of cancer, including stomach<br>• Antiviral qualities protect against flu | Enjoy the many different varieties as a light and refreshing alternative to black tea. Drink without milk. |

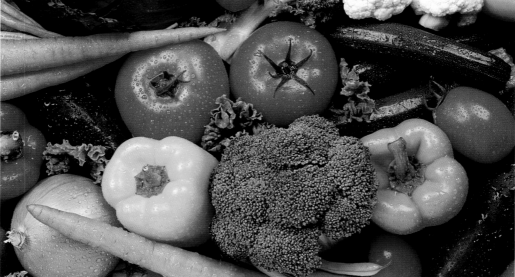

# Exercise plan

Nowadays we spend so much time 'in our heads', and not being active, that exercise is essential in order to bring us back into our bodies and re-establish balance between the physical and mental in our lives.

## BEFORE YOU BEGIN

If you have recently given birth, have been inactive for several years or suffer from any of the medical conditions listed below, then you should, for your own safety, consider making an appointment to see your G.P. before beginning an exercise routine.

- High blood pressure
- Heart trouble
- Family history of early stroke or heart attacks
- Frequent dizzy spells
- Extreme breathlessness after mild exertion
- Arthritis or other bone problems
- Severe muscular, ligament or tendon problems
- Other known or suspected disease

Even in the short term, committing ourselves to a programme of regular exercise can drastically improve our fitness levels. It can – surprisingly quickly, – tone and strengthen our muscles; increase our vitality; reduce insomnia; focus our minds and improve our ability to think clearly; regulate our appetite and encourage us to eat healthily; improve our circulation, breathing, posture, strength, flexibility and stamina; and lift our mood and reduce stress. In the long term, our muscles become more toned, we reduce our risk of disease, improve the way our bodies look and feel, and slow down the ageing process.

## Reasons for not exercising

- **Lack of time**  If you really want to do something you will make time for it.  Besides which you don't have to take part in a marathon or go jogging - exercising can amount to a brisk walk, playing a sport you enjoy, doing some gentle workout exercises at home or even gardening. Try to do some form of exercise daily or at least on a regular basis to achieve the maximum benefit and for the quickest results.

- **No local gym**  There's no need to enrol in a gym, especially as membership can be quite expensive. You could buy a keep fit video or go for a swim at your local pool. Swimming pools and leisure centres also frequently run exercise classes, such as circuit training, yoga and 'hips, bums and tums' sessions that are fun and sociable to attend and also provide a good venue for meeting people and making new friends.

- **Boredom**  This is a popular excuse or is it just an excuse for opting out? There are lots of ways you can make exercising more fun – exercise at different times of the day, try out new sports or classes, ask a friend to join in or workout at home to some music.

- **Absence of results**  Set yourself small goals and keep a diary recording what you have achieved and how you feel. You will then spot those small changes that may otherwise have gone unnoticed.

# Top 50 Superfoods

| FOOD | NUTRIENTS | BENEFITS | SERVING IDEAS |
|------|-----------|----------|---------------|
| **Basil** | • Trace calcium, magnesium and manganese | • Aids digestion and helps relieve colic and wind<br>• Rub basil leaves on insect bites to soothe irritation and prevent infection<br>• Believed to help clear the mind<br>• Stimulates appetite and counteracts nausea | Wonderful flavouring for salads, omelettes, pasta dishes and sauces, combining especially well with tomatoes, eggs, summer vegetables, fish and chicken. Use to make a fresh home-made pesto with olive oil, Parmesan and pine nuts. |
| **Parsley** | • Iron<br>• Vitamins A & C<br>• Calcium<br>• Potassium | • Diuretic and blood purifier<br>• Helps eliminate uric acid, benefiting sufferers of gout and rheumatism<br>• Counters anaemia | Chop and toss generously into salads, rice dishes, soups and casseroles. |
| **Garlic** | • Sulphur<br>• Quercetin (an antioxidant) | • Wonder food with anti-cancer, antiviral, antibacterial and antifungal qualities<br>• Protects the heart by helping to reduce blood cholesterol levels and blood pressure; prevents blood clots by thinning the blood<br>• Good for sinus and chest infections, colds and flu<br>• Can help diabetics by reducing blood sugar levels | Add crushed or finely chopped to dips, salad dressings or stir-fries or as whole cloves with vegetables for roasting. |
| **Ginger** | • Potassium<br>• Calcium<br>• Iron<br>• Magnesium | • Aids digestion and is an effective remedy for nausea<br>• Effective against colds, flu and chest congestion<br>• Reduces the risk of blood clots<br>• Stimulates circulation and cleanses the system | A great flavouring to use in stir-fries and curries, combining well with all kinds of meat, fish and vegetables. |

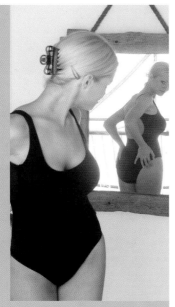

Have you striven for years to attain a well-toned, flat stomach? Do you take a backward glance at your rear end in a shop mirror and cringe at the shape of it? Have you developed thunder thighs? If so, don't worry. The good news is that with time, effort and determination you can do something about it with a combined programme of exercise and healthy eating. But first, it's important to understand how and why these problem areas develop.

## What causes that extra weight?

Hormones, lack of exercise, sluggish circulation, preparation for child-bearing years – all these play a part in the reason why women are predisposed to carrying the body's fat stores in the hip and thigh areas.

The monthly cycle, trapped wind and bloating may also be reasons for a flabby stomach. Plus of course, age, stress, a sedentary lifestyle, lack of exercise and even bad posture can be responsible for extra flesh gained around the abdominal area, hips and buttocks. So let's look at some of these reasons in more detail and what you can do to remedy them.

This excess fat takes some effort to shift because once those fat cells have been formed, although they may shrink in size, they can soon expand in volume and increase in number again. It's therefore important to realise that a lifestyle built around regular exercise and healthy eating needs to be maintained and not just seen as a quick fix followed by a return to lazy and unhealthy ways.

## Lack of exercise

You must give up feeble excuses such as you haven't time, you are too busy or that you have something better to do. In Western societies, we tend to work in largely sedentary jobs then leisure activities- watching T.V, going to the cinemas, reading the paper, sitting in pubs and restaurants, also encourage us to sit around rather than getting us to move. In fact our lifestyles tend to be pretty lazy so we need to make a conscious effort to make time for regular exercise and to be generally more active. If you don't work your muscles, they will turn flabby, but once they are regularly exercised, toned and strengthened, they respond in no time.

**Thousands of women complain about their stomach or backside either being too large or out of shape. But why bemoan the fact that you no longer have the slender buttocks or flat stomach of an eighteen year old? Be honest – you'll never see eighteen again, so isn't it time you stopped wishing and started doing something positive. You may never be a teenager again but that doesn't mean to say you can't restore your figure to a well-toned, lean shape.**

# Top 50 superfoods

| FOOD | NUTRIENTS | BENEFITS | SERVING IDEAS |
|---|---|---|---|
| **Alfalfa** | • Vitamins A & D<br>• Complete protein<br>• Calcium & phosphorus<br>• Iron<br>• Potassium | • One of the most nutritionally rich foods, valued for its ability to cleanse and rejuvenate the system<br>• Anti-inflammatory and aids digestion<br>• Boosts the immune system and relieves arthritis, rheumatism and bloating | Best eaten raw in salads and sandwiches. |
| **Nuts** | • B Vitamins<br>• Vitamin E<br>• Magnesium & manganese<br>• Zinc<br>• Iron<br>• Selenium<br>• Potassium | • Essential fatty acids (found especially in walnuts, almonds and hazelnuts) may protect against heart disease and reduce the risk of strokes. Also vital for tissue development and growth<br>• Vitamin E content reduces the risk of certain cancers | Use unsalted varieties chopped (and toasted if liked) in salads, rice dishes, stir-fries or sprinkled on desserts. Chocolate-coated Brazils make a nourishing treat but are very high in fat and calories so watch how many you eat! |
| **Olive Oil** | • Vitamin E<br>• Monounsaturated fat | • Antioxidant properties help to protect against heart disease, effectively reducing blood cholesterol levels<br>• Reduces the risk of certain cancers<br>• Eases arthritis<br>• May help liver and gall bladder problems<br>• Improves digestion | Ideal for salad dressings, marinades, light pan-frying and for drizzling on vegetables for roasting, but use in moderation as like all fats and oils, it's high in calories. |
| **Seeds** | • Vitamin E<br>• Omega-6 fatty acids<br>• Iron<br>• Zinc<br>• Fibre<br>• Potassium | • Vitamin E (especially high in sunflower seeds) protects cells from oxidation, improves circulation and normal blood clotting<br>• Reduces risk of heart disease and strokes by lowering blood cholesterol<br>• Pumpkin seeds promote good prostate health<br>• Supports the immune system and has restorative qualities | Pumpkin, sunflower and sesame seeds can all be scattered on salads, vegetable dishes, cereals and soups or on home-made breads and puddings. |

# Why and where flab settles

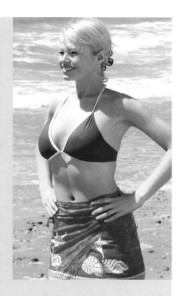

By the end of three weeks, with perseverance and dedication, you will:

- Feel healthier
- Feel more confident
- Feel much better about how you look in snug-fitting clothes
- Want to wear cropped tops
- Have improved posture

No more excuses about starting tomorrow or next week, there is no time like today! So start planning now and get working towards your dream of achieving your perfect dress size.

## Your age

It is a pity that so much attention nowadays is focused upon the way a woman looks and the changes caused by ageing, especially when you are over 30.

In truth this is the age when a woman's metabolism naturally slows down, because the body has reached a turning point when nature is equipping it with extra baggage, generally in the shape of excess flesh around the waist, thighs and upper arms. The only remedy is to accept these changes gracefully, but at the same time to fight back.

### In Your Twenties

This is when many of us end up sitting at a desk for 6-7 hours a day. Unfortunately it is also the time when the mind is stimulated but not the buttocks, so make sure they don't turn flabby. You need to integrate some cardiovascular exercising, especially those directed towards the gluteal region, i.e. step classes, brisk walking, skipping and running.

### In Your Thirties

A time in life when many women have their children, resulting in flabby stomach muscles that need a little more exercising than breathing in. If you don't work on this area, the muscles will just remain lazy and flabby. Remember to ask your health visitor for advice if you've recently had a baby.

### In Your Forties

This is the time when muscles in the backs of the arms may begin to follow gravity. To counteract this problem and tone up the muscles, it is important to start exercising the shoulders and arms.

### In Your Fifties

Although active when younger, with the passing of years, motivating one's legs to go for a long walk can get harder, but any type of cardiovascular exercise will remedy this. Try dancing or brisk walking and remember you're never too old to take up cycling.

# Top 50 superfoods

| FOOD | NUTRIENTS | BENEFITS | SERVING IDEAS |
|------|-----------|----------|---------------|
| Shellfish | • Vitamin B12<br>• Selenium<br>• Iodine & zinc<br>• Phosphorus<br>• Iron | • Maintains the nervous system and regulates metabolism<br>• Helps to reduce the risk of some cancers and protects against heart disease and circulation problems<br>• Strengthens the immune system<br>• Known as an aphrodisiac<br>• Anti-inflammatory benefits | Use for curries, fish pies, pasta, dishes, stir-fries, kebabs, sauces and classics like Paella. |
| Egg | • Iron<br>• B vitamins<br>• Vitamins A & E<br>• Selenium<br>• Zinc<br>• Good source of protein | • Antioxidant qualities may help to protect against some forms of cancer<br>• One of the few sources of vitamin B12 – essential for the nervous system – for vegetarians | Poach, boil, bake, scramble or use to make an omelette or soufflé. Wonderfully versatile for all kinds of quick meals and partner well with cheese, tomatoes, bacon, smoked salmon, watercress and spinach. |
| Milk | • Vitamin A<br>• B vitamins<br>• Calcium<br>• Zinc<br>• Phosphorous<br>• Good source of protein | • Rich source of easily absorbed calcium, essential for strong teeth and bones.<br>• Contains a range of other minerals and vitamins and considered a perfect food.<br>• Skimmed and semi-skimmed milks are very low in fat, and although fat-soluble vitamins A and D are lost, they have a slightly higher calcium content than whole (full-fat) milk. | Use skimmed or semi-skimmed milk in hot drinks and for sweet and savoury sauces, fruit smoothies, pancakes and milk puddings. |
| Yogurt | • Calcium<br>• B vitamins<br>• Phosphorus | • The 'good' bacteria in live yogurt suppresses harmful bacteria in the gut, so aiding digestion and relieving gastrointestinal problems<br>• Restores intestinal flora if consumed after a course of antibiotics<br>• Can protect against thrush<br>• May reduce the risk of colon cancer | Delicious with a compote of fresh or dried fruits or on breakfast cereals but also use for making salad dressings, dips, and marinades and raita to serve with curry. |

# Why and where flab settles

## Bloating

The 'time of the month' plays havoc not only with emotions but also body shape, sometimes making you feel that you look like a beached whale! The hormone progesterone is the guilty party. Generally a week before the onset of your period, the body begins to produce extra progesterone (the hormone responsible for causing fluid retention) in preparation for an egg to be fertilized. Naturally this fluid manifests itself around the stomach. Once the 'all-clear' signal is heard and the body knows that it is not pregnant, progesterone levels drop to their normal level, excess fluid is released through your urine, and the stomach returns to its normal shape.

It is during this difficult build-up period that your mind often plays tricks on you. The raised levels of progesterone can affect one's mood and body image, so although rationally you know you aren't any fatter, you still feel that you are.

## Trapped wind

The human body is an amazing organism but there are times when it refuses to accept quietly the foods it is being fed and reacts in unpredictable ways. Many find certain foods, such as pulses, Brussels sprouts and cabbage cause over production of wind in the digestive system resulting in a feeling of fullness and a rather bloated appearance.

The most effective way to deal with this is to monitor your diet and restrict those foods which are responsible.

# Top 50 superfoods

| FOOD | NUTRIENTS | BENEFITS | SERVING IDEAS |
|---|---|---|---|
| Quinoa | • B vitamins (especially B$_6$, niacin and thiamin)<br>• Iron<br>• Calcium<br>• Good source of protein | • Wheat and gluten-free so suitable for coeliacs and anyone allergic to wheat<br>• Offers more potassium and iron than other grains | Cook and use like rice or like cracked (bulghur) wheat in a tabbouleh-style salad, with chopped cucumber, tomato and lots of herbs. |
| Oats | • B Vitamins<br>• Vitamin E<br>• Calcium<br>• Magnesium<br>• Fibre | • Effectively reduces blood cholesterol, increasing beneficial HDL cholesterol levels<br>• Eases constipation<br>• May calm the nerves<br>• Helps stabilize blood sugar levels, so useful for diabetics | Porridge oats or muesli for breakfast make an excellent start to the day. Oats can also be added to crumble toppings, used for making flapjacks or coating rissoles. |
| Rice (brown) | • B vitamins<br>• Fibre<br>• Manganese<br>• Magnesium | • Helps to control blood sugar levels, making it useful for diabetics<br>• May help with psoriasis<br>• Aids digestive disorders and calms the nervous system<br>• Reduces the risk of bowel and colon cancer and also kidney stones | Toss with vegetables, nuts or dried fruits for a tasty accompaniment or to make a rice salad, or with meat, fish and poultry for a pilaf, biryani or Jambalaya. Also good for stuffing vegetables. |
| Oily Fish | • Omega-3 essential fatty acids<br>• Vitamins A & D<br>• Iodine<br>• Phosphorus<br>• Selenium | • Essential for healthy cell function, reduces blood cholesterol levels, blood pressure and likelihood of blood clots, lowering the risk of heart disease and strokes<br>• Helps rheumatoid arthritis due to anti-inflammatory properties and may protect against some cancers<br>• Improves circulation and skin disorders such as psoriasis and dermatitis | Include fresh tuna, mackerel, salmon, herrings, anchovies and sardines – bake, grill or barbecue. |

## MOTHERHOOD

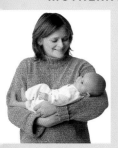

It is, of course, normal to put on weight during pregnancy. This gain is made up of the weight of the fluid in which the baby lives in the womb, the weight of the baby itself and the weight of the extra fat laid down to provide the energy needed for breast feeding. The average weight gain is in the region of 12.5 kg (27 lb). Breastfeeding then helps to break down this fat but if you choose to bottle feed instead or have put on too much weight during pregnancy, that fat and excess weight will remain. Also during pregnancy, the abdominal muscles are stretched and it's these muscles which maintain your shape and figure. However with exercise even the most flabby muscles can be toned up and restored to good condition.

## Beer Belly

Beer is not the only culprit; in fact any alcoholic drink can increase the size of the stomach simply because every gram of alcohol contains 7 calories, almost twice as much energy as each gram of carbohydrate or protein. So if you know that alcohol is the cause of your flabby stomach, there is only one answer - give up, or cut down, drinking the stuff!

## Stress

Whenever you are worried or under stress, the body reacts. Some people find that the stomach is particularly affected when it is suddenly bombarded with large amounts of the stress hormone cortisol. Because the stomach area has more receptors than any other part of the body, the hormone is automatically pumped into the fat cells lying around the waist where it settles.

In order to deal with stress and to reduce the effect it has on your stomach, there are several positive things you can do:

- Learn to relax
- Take regular exercise
- Practise deep breathing
- Have a good laugh
- If you drink or smoke, cut down

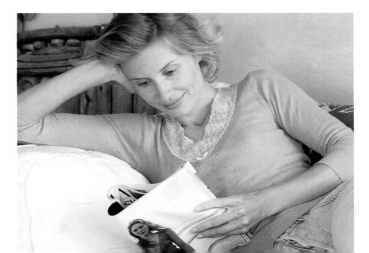

| FOOD | NUTRIENTS | BENEFITS | SERVING IDEAS |
|---|---|---|---|
| Pepper (sweet) | • Vitamins C & E<br>• Beta-carotene<br>• Iron<br>• Potassium<br>• Bioflavonoids | • High antioxidant properties, known to reduce the risk of heart disease, strokes, cataracts and some forms of cancer<br>• Good for skin and bones | Wonderfully colourful used for salads, stir-fries and for stuffing whole. |
| Lentils | • B vitamins<br>• Fibre<br>• Iron<br>• Potassium<br>• Selenium<br>• Good source of protein | • Reduces blood cholesterol levels and regulates high blood pressure, protecting against heart disease<br>• Aids functioning of bowels and colon<br>• Fibre helps to control blood sugar levels<br>• Fights fatigue, anaemia and poor memory | Excellent for making curries, soups and vegetarian patties or adding to casseroles. Green Puy lentils are good in a salad or braised with sausages. |
| Pulses | • B vitamins<br>• Iron<br>• Folate<br>• Potassium<br>• Fibre<br>• Manganese<br>• Good source of protein | • Lowers blood cholesterol levels by about 20 per cent if eaten regularly, reducing the risk of heart disease and strokes<br>• Helps to control blood sugar levels, so valuable for diabetics<br>• Reduces blood pressure<br>• Helps anaemia | All kinds of beans (and lentils) make fabulous casseroles, soups, salads, curries and vegetarian loaves and rissoles. |
| Soya Bean | • Complete protein<br>• B vitamins<br>• Iron<br>• Folate & calcium<br>• Potassium<br>• Fibre | • Contain phytoestrogens, known to protect against cancer of the breast, prostate and colon. Helps to balance hormone levels<br>• Reduces the risk of osteoporosis<br>• Reduces blood cholesterol levels and blood pressure<br>• Eases constipation<br>• Regulates blood sugar levels | Add beans to soups and casseroles but also enjoy soya products such as T.V.P, used as a meat substitute and tofu (soya bean curd). |

# Get moving

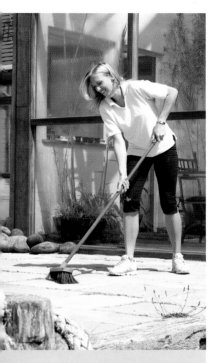

Exercise is the ideal way to get the body system going, increasing the metabolic rate and for improving muscle tone. Sports are good but there is also a lot you can do just around the home and at work to build up your level of activity.

## At home

**HOUSEWORK:** It's official – a vigorous burst of housework can be as good for you as a trip to the gym. All those mundane jobs such as vacuuming, dusting, sweeping, ironing and cleaning windows are all good forms of exercise and help to burn calories as well as tone muscles. So rather than seeing the housework as a boring chore, think of it as an opportunity for a regular exercise routine. Naturally the harder you work at it, the more calories you burn and the better the results – both physically and

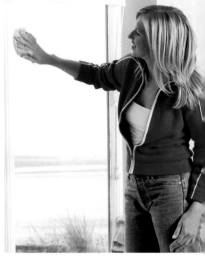

aesthetically! You might even give the house a good spring-clean and apart from benefiting from the exercise, you'll also be rewarded with a fresh and sparkling home to enjoy and a great feeling of satisfaction.

- Vacuuming can burn up 6 calories a minute

- Climbing the stairs burns 10 calories a minute

- One hour's worth of digging in the garden can burn up 392 calories

- Scrubbing the floor burns up 400 calories an hour

**GARDENING:** If you have a garden, then look no further for regular exercise. Mowing the lawn is great for toning up the abdominal muscles; how about pruning those high branches – no better exercise for toning the arms and back; or pull up weeds – it's the ideal answer for working on those thighs as you bend and straighten. It also helps to tone up buttocks and arms and the bonus is that your garden will look great too.

# Top 50 superfoods

| FOOD | NUTRIENTS | BENEFITS | SERVING IDEAS |
|------|-----------|----------|---------------|
| Carrot | • Beta-carotene<br>• Fibre<br>• Potassium | • May help protect against cancer<br>• Excellent detoxifier, cleansing and nourishing every system of the body<br>• Promotes healthy vision, skin and bones<br>• Aids the respiratory and digestive system and helps ward off colds<br>• Reduces the risk of heart disease and strokes | Delicious raw, grated in a salad or cut into chunky sticks as crudités. Serve boiled, steamed or braised or add to soups and casseroles. Also fab used to make a moist carrot cake for a special treat. |
| Pea | • Vitamin C<br>• Thiamin (vitamin B$_1$)<br>• Fibre<br>• Folate<br>• Iron<br>• Zinc | • Helps to reduce blood cholesterol levels, reducing the risk of heart disease<br>• Fibre helps to steady blood sugar levels | Freshly podded or frozen, they make a popular accompaniment cooked solo with a sprig of fresh mint or tossed with some crisp bacon. Or combine with other vegetables, such as carrots, sweetcorn, mange-tout or spring onions. |
| Sweet Potato | • Beta-carotene<br>• Vitamins C & E<br>• Potassium<br>• Fibre | • Good for the heart<br>• Reduces the risk of some cancers<br>• Improves condition of the skin<br>• Helps to regulate high blood pressure<br>• Cleanses and detoxifies the system, boosting circulation | Cook as for regular potatoes. Their delicious sweetness makes them ideal for adding to soups, casseroles, pies and puddings. |
| Onion | • Quercetin (antioxidant)<br>• Sulphur | • Reduces the risk of heart disease and strokes, thins the blood and reduces harmful cholesterol levels and protects against some cancers, particularly stomach<br>• Antibacterial and antiviral, helping to fight colds, relieve bronchial congestion, asthma and hayfever<br>• Effective against arthritis, gout and rheumatism | Indispensable for flavouring cooked dishes and salads. Also good stuffed and baked. |

# Get moving

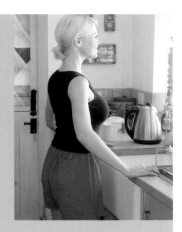

## SPARE MINUTE EXERCISES

Here are two simple exercises that can be done in any spare moment – whilst washing the dishes, waiting in the bus queue, even when serving dinner!

• Buttock clencher: Clench your buttocks, hold for a few seconds and then simply release – perfect for toning up the buttocks.

• Thigh firmer: When waiting for the kettle to boil, gradually raise and lower your leg straight behind and as high as you can, almost like a ballerina. Hold the position for 30 seconds and then repeat with the other leg.

**STAIRS:** Forget about investing in a step machine when you have your very own. Carrying clothes upstairs, bringing laundry down, going upstairs to make the beds, bringing bins down to empty – all are ideal for strengthening and toning leg muscles. You could even just run up and down the stairs a few times daily, not for a specific reason, but just to help exercise those muscles.

**WALKIES:** Take the dog for a 30 minute walk each day – perfect all-round exercise. If you don't have a dog, offer to walk a friend or neighbour's dog. Plenty of dog-owners simply don't have the time or ability to do it themselves and welcome the offer of help. Try advertising in a local newsagent.

**CAR WASHING:** Wash and polish the car manually rather than use a car wash. You could also put the money saved towards that new outfit!

**TOYS & EQUIPMENT:** You can buy various exercise machines to use at home but this doesn't have to be a large or expensive item like an exercise bike or a rowing machine. A mini trampoline doesn't take up much floor space or how about a simple skipping rope? Skipping is the ideal all-over exercise and perfect for stretching the leg muscles. It also works the heart, lungs and upper body to get a really good workout. Play some favourite music and bounce or skip in time with the rhythm.

# Top 50 superfoods

| FOOD | NUTRIENTS | BENEFITS | SERVING IDEAS |
|---|---|---|---|
| **Spinach** | • Beta-carotene<br>• Vitamin C & E<br>• Iron<br>• Calcium & folate<br>• Potassium<br>• Fibre | • Green leafy vegetables help to reduce the risk of cancer of the lung, stomach, prostate, bladder and skin<br>• Rich in antioxidants, reducing the risk of heart disease, cataracts and strokes<br>• Helps to regulate high blood pressure<br>• Fights fatigue and mental strain | Young leaves are good raw for salads. Lightly cooked, spinach makes a delicious addition to savoury tarts, risotto and curries. |
| **Cabbage** | • Vitamins C<br>• Fibre<br>• Beta-carotene<br>• Folate<br>• Potassium<br>• Iron<br>• Magnesium | • Prevents anaemia, protects against stress and infection, and detoxifies the stomach<br>• Anti-carcinogenic cocktail – reduces the risk of stomach, lung, skin, breast, womb and colon cancer<br>• High antioxidant levels reduce the risk of heart disease and strokes | Use shredded, raw, white or red cabbage for making coleslaw. If cooked, cabbage (also spring greens) should be shredded then lightly steamed or stir-fried. Large green leaves can be used for wrapping round savoury mixtures to make parcels. |
| **Broccoli** | • Vitamin C<br>• Beta-carotene<br>• Folate<br>• Iron & zinc<br>• Potassium<br>• Calcium | • Protects against cancer of the lung, colon and breast<br>• Inhibits the spread of certain cancers<br>• High in antioxidants, so helps to reduce the risk of heart disease and strokes<br>• Antibacterial and antiviral | Lightly steam or stir-fry or cut into small florets and use raw in salads or to serve as crudités. Also makes a good soup. |
| **Watercress** | • Beta-carotene<br>• Vitamin C & E<br>• Vitamin B6<br>• Folate<br>• Iron<br>• Potassium<br>• Zinc<br>• Calcium | • Part of the cancer-fighting cruciferous family, effective against cancers of the colon, rectum and bladder<br>• Rich in antioxidants, helps to protect against heart disease and strokes<br>• A natural antibiotic, boosting the immune system, helps relieve stomach and respiratory problems and purifies the system<br>• Stimulates circulation | Add to salads, soups and sandwiches or use to make a tasty dip with reduced-fat Greek-style yogurt. |

# Get moving

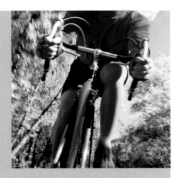

Exercise is good for you and should also be fun but there are simple steps you can make to build exercise into your daily lifestyle. For example, if you only have a short journey to work, consider cycling or walking some days rather than driving or using public transport.

## At work

Those who are employed in office jobs and spend all day sitting at a desk are more prone to the development of cellulite due to an overall sluggish circulation, especially in the buttocks and thigh areas. Try to get up every hour or so and have a walk around, even if it's just a visit to the loo! And at lunchtime, make sure you go out for walk. If you work in an office with several floors, always take the stairs rather than the lift. There are also many ways of including exercise into your journey to work.

- If you only have a short journey, consider cycling or walking some days rather than driving.
- If you travel by bus, alight a stop or two early and walk the extra distance instead.
- If you leave the car in a car park, park it at the far end so as to walk a little further to your destination.
- If you use an underground station, take the stairs rather than the escalator or at least walk up the escalator, rather than just standing in line while you're carried to the top.

## IF YOU HAVEN'T EXERCISED FOR A WHILE:

- Don't exercise too strenuously to begin with – overtired muscles create waste products and put a strain on the lymphatic system

- Whatever exercise you decide to do, begin slowly and then build up gradually

- Don't push yourself too hard

- Try to find an exercise that frees the mind

- Don't choose something you don't like – remember exercise should be enjoyable

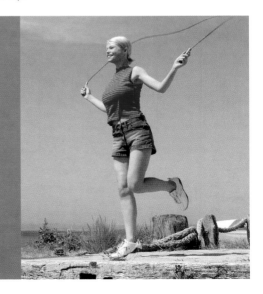

# Top 50 superfoods

| FOOD | NUTRIENTS | BENEFITS | SERVING IDEAS |
|---|---|---|---|
| Asparagus | • Beta-carotene<br>• Folate<br>• Fibre<br>• Vitamin C<br>• Vitamin E | • Diuretic and mildly laxative<br>• Good for the kidneys, liver, skin and bones<br>• Contains the antioxidant glutathione, said to prevent the formation of cataracts | Perfect for stir-fries, omelettes, savoury tarts and salads and makes a delicious soup. |
| Beetroot | • Vitamins C<br>• Iron<br>• Potassium<br>• Folate | • General tonic; supports the immune system<br>• Detoxifies the liver, gall bladder and kidneys<br>• Maintains normal blood pressure and combats anaemia | Go for raw or cooked beetroot, but not the type pickled in vinegar, and use grated or diced in salads and relishes. |
| Avocado | • Good source of monounsaturated fats<br>• Vitamins B & E<br>• Selenium<br>• Beta-carotene<br>• Potassium | • Improves condition of skin and hair<br>• Soothes digestive tract<br>• Good for anaemia<br>• Beneficial fats help to reduce blood cholesterol<br>• Helps stress and depression | Delicious as a light meal with prawns, smoked salmon or tomatoes or used for a sandwich filling, salad or dip (such as Guacamole). |
| Tomato | • Vitamins C & E<br>• Beta-carotene<br>• Potassium | • Contains the bioflavonoid lycopene, said to prevent some forms of cancer, particularly prostate<br>• Antioxidant properties reduce the risk of heart disease, strokes and cataracts<br>• Cooking enhances some of the health-giving qualities of tomatoes, particularly the effectiveness of lycopene | Lovely for salads and salsas, grilled on toast or as part of a healthy cooked breakfast. Also add to curries, soups, casseroles and risottos. |

# Get sporty

The golden rules of exercise are to start gently, to build gradually, and to do it regularly. To be effective, you need to aim for three to four sessions per week of at least 20 minutes each time. Varying your activity will help to keep you motivated and make exercise more fun. There are all kinds of options so check out your local fitness and leisure centres and sports clubs as well as finding out what evening or weekend classes are offered at schools in your area. Get a friend or your partner to join a class or take up a sport with you to encourage each other and add to the enjoyment.

## Pedal power

Cycling is an excellent all-round exercise for firming and toning the fronts and backs of your thighs, the abdomen and buttocks. It will also improve your strength and stamina. You can cycle as speedily, or as sedately as you like and your bike can be any style that you feel comfortable riding. A bicycle ride in the open air can also lift your mood and act as an enjoyable way of seeing the countryside as well as being a fun activity to enjoy with family or friends. And if you live within a few miles of work, take to your wheels instead of using the car or public transport. Apart from the exercise benefits, you'll be helping to reduce pollution levels by choosing the 'green' alternative.

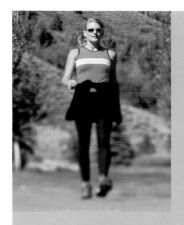

**CALORIE COUNTER**
Different kinds of exercise burn up various amounts of calories:

Walking: if done for 30 minutes burns up 230 calories

Cycling: if done for 30 minutes burns up 190 calories

Swimming: if done for 20 minutes burns up 180 calories

Skating: if done for 20 minutes burns up 205 calories

Dancing: if done for 25 minutes burns up 215 calories

Aerobics: if done for an hour burns up 305 calories

(All values are approximate)

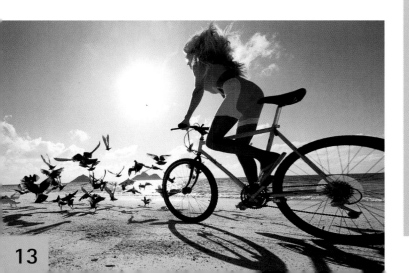

| FOOD | NUTRIENTS | BENEFITS | SERVING IDEAS |
|------|-----------|----------|---------------|
| Kiwi Fruit | • Vitamin C<br>• Vitamin E<br>• Potassium<br>• Fibre | • Excellent source of vitamin C. A single fruit provides the full adult daily requirement.<br>• Potassium helps to regulate the body fluid levels and to ensure healthy blood pressure and a steady heartbeat.<br>• Good for the digestion with laxative properties.<br>• May help alleviate depression. | Easy to eat – just cut like a boiled egg and scoop with a teaspoon. Lovely in fruit salads and partners well with ham, smoked fish and chicken. |
| Mango | • Vitamin C<br>• Beta-carotene | • Carotenes act as antioxidants and help to protect against heart disease and cancer. May help, in particular, to protect against cervical cancer.<br>• Vitamin C also acts as an antioxidant. One medium-size fruit supplies more than the adult daily requirement. | Slice mango (and papaya) into tropical fruit salads. Delicious blended in a smoothie for a nourishing breakfast in a glass. |
| Prunes | • Vitamin B6<br>• Iron<br>• Potassium<br>• Fibre | • The mineral iron helps to carry oxygen around the body<br>• Fibre helps to maintain a healthy digestive system.<br>• Effective natural laxative.<br>• Good for reducing blood cholesterol.<br>• Good ability to absorb damaged free radicals, helping to fight off cancer. | Delicious in a breakfast compote and they also combine well with meat dishes, especially with pork. Prunes wrapped in lean bacon and grilled make a popular party nibble. |
| Dates | • Vitamin C<br>• Potassium<br>• Fibre<br>• Iron | • Gentle laxative<br>• Energizing and nourishing fruit, useful for convalescents | Delicious served with a tasty cheese as a simple dessert or fill with soft cheese for a party nibble. They can also be chopped and added to salads or North African-style casseroles or included in a homemade date and walnut loaf. |

# Get sporty

## Take a hike

According to experts, you don't have to work up a sweat at the gym on a workout to tone your muscles – a brisk walk is just as good. In fact the medical profession agrees that the health benefits associated with walking exceed those of every other form of exercise. What better all-round form of exercise could you ask for? If you can, choose to walk in a pleasant, traffic-free environment, like a park, but not somewhere lonely or after dark, if walking on your own.

To get the full benefit, aim to do three or four 20-minute sessions of brisk walking a week. You should be able to cover a mile in about 15 minutes. The technique is simple: shoulders back, neck relaxed, shoulders aligned directly above your hips and a heel-toe roll in a straight line, through the foot, narrowing the width of your track to allow for greater speed with arms and legs moving in sync. Slow down if you get out of breath – you should be going at a pace where you're still able to chat. Each week, try to improve on your efforts by going a little further. Walking is a great way to relieve stress and if you have children and find it difficult to make time for other forms of exercise, take a picnic and turn your walk into a family outing. Alternatively for group walks, you might like to consider joining the Ramblers Association.

### POWER WALKING CAN:
- lower cholesterol
- relieve chronic pain
- regulate blood pressure
- alleviate depression
- help insomnia and infertility

### TIPS
- Exercise until pleasantly tired, but don't push yourself to exhaustion. The right level will leave you slightly breathless but not feeling ready to collapse.

- Always warm-up before exercising to prepare your muscles and keep your joints fully flexible. This could just be some gentle running on the spot and some stretching.

- It's also important to gently wind down your exercise session, especially following vigorous exercise. This will help to avoid muscle strain or injury.

- Don't start exercising immediately after a heavy meal. Allow about 1 hour before starting.

- If you feel faint or dizzy, out of breath or experience any pain, stop immediately and take a rest – you might be doing too much too soon.

- Always dress in comfortable clothing that allows you to move freely and be sure to wear a good pair of trainers with good arch support and a thick cushioned sole.

- Think of exercise as a natural, essential part of your life – just like eating or sleeping.

| FOOD | NUTRIENTS | BENEFITS | SERVING IDEAS |
|---|---|---|---|
| Grapefruit | • Vitamin C<br>• Potassium<br>• Beta-carotene (in pink variety)<br>• Bioflavonoids | • High vitamin C content (especially in pink variety) helps fight infections<br>• Bioflavonoids may help protect against certain forms of cancer.<br>• Beta-carotene is essential for growth, vision and immune function | Makes a refreshing low-fat, low-calorie breakfast (if not sprinkled with sugar). Pink-fleshed varieties taste sweeter than the yellow type. The sharp flavour also marries well with tangy cheese, Parma ham, smoked fish and shellfish in salads. |
| Orange | • Vitamin C<br>• Bioflavonoids<br>• Folate<br>• Potassium | • High vitamin C content helps to protect against many forms of cancer, particularly stomach and oesophagus<br>• Protects against heart attacks and strokes, reducing blood cholesterol levels<br>• Boosts immune system and fights colds and flu | Enjoy as an anytime snack or segment and add to salads. Also useful for making tangy sauces and marinades. |
| Pineapple | • Potassium | • Contains the enzyme bromelain which has anti-inflammatory and antibacterial properties<br>• Relieves arthritis<br>• Aids digestion and improves circulation<br>• May help angina | Add in chunks to a chicken curry, toss into a sweet and sour stir-fry or use to make a great salsa to serve with ham. Also delicious thickly sliced and sprinkled with liqueur. |
| Grapes | • Potassium<br>• Fibre<br>• Quercetin (an antioxidant) | • Powerful antioxidant flavonoids help protect against heart disease and certain cancers<br>• Powerful detoxifier, so improves the condition of the skin<br>• Treats gout as well as liver and kidney disorders<br>• Nourishing and strengthening qualities make grapes useful for convalescents as well as those with fatigue and anaemia | Eat as they are or add to fruit salads or a fruit jelly. |

# Get sporty

## Pick up a racket

Tennis is a brilliant exercise for promoting shapely legs. Remember, it's never too late to start so if you're a complete beginner, find out about coaching classes at your local fitness centre or tennis club. Singles tends to be a more energetic game than doubles but play with others of a similar standard so you don't over-exert yourself. Tennis is an excellent way to improve strength, stamina and flexibility and co-ordination. It also provides a good mental workout. Other racket sports include squash and badminton. All provide good aerobic exercise, help to build stronger muscles and improve posture and are efficient at burning calories.

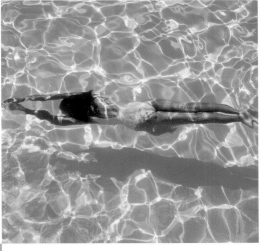

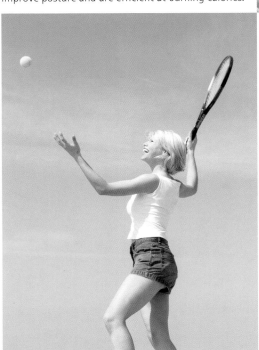

## Make a splash

If you exercise in water, it is 15 times more effective than doing the same exercise on land simply because of the resistance against your muscles. Water is a superb and quick way to tone your body because whichever direction you move, your body will still have to push against the water. Regular lane-swimming is excellent exercise or you might like to enrol in water-fitness classes, such as aqua fitness, water Pilates, aqua combat or even aqua jogging – check out what's available at your local pools.

There are also often ladies only sessions and crèche facilities for parents with young children, leaving you free to take to the water. Swim with a smooth, easy relaxed stroke and concentrate on a good stretch and streamlined body position. Try a variety of styles – breaststroke, backstroke etc, that way you exercise different groups of muscles and joints.

# Top 50 superfoods

| FOOD | NUTRIENTS | BENEFITS | SERVING IDEAS |
|---|---|---|---|
| **Cranberry** | • Vitamin C<br>• Beta-carotene<br>• Potassium<br>• Iron | • Helps prevent and treat urinary tract infections, particularly cystitis<br>• Antifungal, antibacterial and antiviral<br>• May help people with kidney stones | Enjoy as a breakfast juice or in cocktails. Cooked berries go well with meat, poultry and game dishes or can be braised or stir-fried with red cabbage. |
| **Blueberry** | • Vitamin C<br>• Fibre | • Helps combat cystitis and other urinary tract infections<br>• Detoxifier and antioxidant with anti-infection and anti-inflammatory properties<br>• Benefits eyesight; may improve night and light vision; prevent cataracts<br>• Memory enhancer<br>• Improves circulation, helping to prevent broken and varicose veins | Delicious raw for a fruity snack, added to a fruit salad or scattered on desserts and breakfast cereals. Popular for including in homemade muffins. |
| **Raspberries** | • Vitamin C<br>• Potassium<br>• Folate<br>• Fibre | • Excellent source of vitamin C, which acts as an antioxidant in the body and helps to protect against heart disease and cancer.<br>• Higher in fibre than many other fruits. | A nutritious low-calorie choice for a dessert. Combine with other berries or serve piled in a seeded melon. Use to fill a sponge cake or to make a sauce for ice-cream for a special treat. |
| **Strawberries** | • Vitamin C<br>• Beta-carotene<br>• Potassium<br>• Folate | • Excellent source of vitamin C<br>• Anti-cancer, antiviral and antibacterial qualities. | Simply delicious on their own or combined with other summer fruits. They also blend well in a smoothie, make great ice-cream and combine well with avocado in a salad. |

# Get sporty

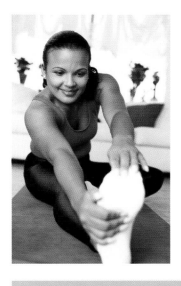

## Join a class

There is a wide range of classes available for all ages and all levels of fitness at gyms, leisure centres and adult education centres. Aerobics and keep fit classes combine jogging and jumping movements with stretch and strength exercises to give you an all-over workout that strengthens and tones the legs as well as the rest of the body. Step aerobics helps to sculpt the legs but make sure you don't do more than one class a week otherwise you will risk bulking up your legs too much.

## Get in the swing

It's surprising how far golfers walk in pursuit of that little white ball – usually a few miles in every round! For maximum benefit, don't dawdle. Choose a time when the course is fairly quiet and there are not too many other players around and stride out after each shot.

## IDEAS FOR ACTIVITIES

Now you are becoming more and more active you might like to think of taking up further activities. Don't get caught up in what you think you 'ought' to do, though: remember, it is supposed to be fun, so choose something that inspires you. Maybe there's something you've always longed to do but never previously had the opportunity? Now's your chance – remember, it's never too late...

- Abseiling
- Athletics
- Baseball, softball
- Basketball
- Body combat
- Boxing
- Cheerleading
- Circus skills
- Cricket
- Dance (ballet, line dancing, Latin, ballroom, jive, hip-hop, street, jazz, ceroc)
- Dance combat
- Diving
- Football
- Hang gliding
- Horseriding
- Ice-skating
- Martial arts (karate, tai quando, aikido)
- Pilates
- Pot-holing
- Rock climbing
- Skiing
- Synchro-swimming
- Tai chi
- Trampolining
- Volleyball
- Watersports (canoeing, rowing, sailing, water-skiing, body-surfing, scuba diving, wind-surfing)
- Yoga

# Top 50 superfoods

Include these superhealthy foods in your diet. Not only are they bursting with nutrients and will help you achieve your desired weight and figure but they will promote tip-top health too.

| FOOD | NUTRIENTS | BENEFITS | SERVING IDEAS |
|---|---|---|---|
| **Banana** | • Potassium<br>• Fibre<br>• Folate<br>• Vitamin B6 | • Rich in the amino acid, tryptophan, known to lift the spirits and aid sleep<br>• Aids functioning of cells, nerves and muscles<br>• Eases high blood pressure<br>• Boosts energy levels<br>• Soothes the stomach and digestive system, relieving both constipation and diarrhoea<br>• Helps the body eliminate toxins | Perfect for a quick breakfast or snack on the run, providing a substantial energy boost. Also good sliced on cereal or porridge, mashed in a sandwich or blended in a smoothie with semi-skimmed milk and low-fat yogurt. |
| **Apricot** | • Beta-carotene<br>• Iron (particularly when dried)<br>• Potassium | • Antioxidant qualities may help to reduce risk of heart disease and certain cancers<br>• Laxative<br>• Helps prevent high blood pressure and fight fatigue<br>• May help to prevent osteoporosis | Dried apricots make a healthy snack or add them to home-made muesli, fruit compotes, rice dishes and casseroles. Poached fresh apricots make a delicious dessert, served with reduced-fat Greek-style yogurt. |
| **Apple** | • Vitamin C<br>• Potassium<br>• Fibre | • Removes impurities in the liver<br>• Aids digestion and encourages natural beneficial bacteria to thrive in the digestive tract<br>• Good for skin, rheumatism, circulation and arthritis if eaten regularly<br>• Effective detoxifier and pick-me-up | A popular snack or slice and add to salads. Cooking apples are delicious stewed or stuffed and baked. |
| **Blackcurrant** | • Vitamin C<br>• Vitamin E<br>• Fibre<br>• Potassium | • Contains pigments called anthocyanins, which are anti-inflammatory and antibacterial<br>• Soothes sore throats<br>• Eases stomach upsets<br>• Antioxidant qualities help to protect against heart disease, strokes and certain cancers | Mix with other currants and red berries to make a lovely fruit compote or filling for a Summer Pudding. Also good for making home-made jam, sauce for ice-cream or cordial. |

# Body contouring & toning exercises

As well as including regular aerobic activities in your lifestyle, such as cycling, walking and swimming that will help to burn fat, to get that figure you want, you also need to do toning and strengthening exercises to build up specific muscle groups.

There are exercises to help tone up particular parts of the body (see *spot reducing for problem* areas on pages 25-31) but to begin with, you need an all-round, whole body exercise routine. Start by doing 10 -15 minutes each day, and aim to build up to about 20 minutes. Alternatively you may prefer to do slightly longer sessions on alternate days or 3-4 days a week but whatever programme suits your lifestyle, make sure it is a regular routine and not just the occasional burst. Of course you can join a gym or class for regular sessions but alternatively, find a convenient time to fit in this workout at home.

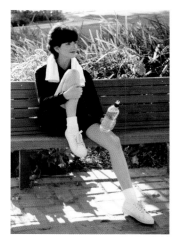

## GUIDELINES

- Choose a time that's convenient for you and mark it in your diary. This may be before or after work, although preferably not late at night, when you're likely to be tired. If you have young children, make time to exercise when they are at school or playgroup.
- Do not exercise immediately after eating a meal. Leave a gap of at least 1 hour.
- Wear loose comfortable clothing so your skin can breathe and sweat is carried from the surface of the skin.
- Choose a light and airy room (or even the garden) to exercise in with plenty room to stretch out. Use a workout mat if the floor isn't carpeted or lay the mat on the grass outside.
- Drink plenty of water during and after exercising.

- You can exercise to music as long as the rhythm is in keeping with the timing of the movements and doesn't force you to do them too quickly.
- Start slowly and build up the routine at your own pace. Remember it's the quality of the movements that counts, not the quantity, so focus on perfecting the technique.
- Do not get up too quickly after exercising lying down, to avoid the possibility of dizziness.
- Aim to spend about 30 seconds on each exercise on each side (when worked separately). As you become fitter, you can gradually increase this time to first 40 seconds then up to 1 minute for each exercise.
- Take a health check with your G.P to confirm that you are fit and well before starting any exercise programme.

## FREE FOODS

**Eat as much as you like of these:**

- Bean sprouts
- Broccoli
- Celery
- Cucumber
- Fennel
- Spinach and other green leafy vegetables
- Tomatoes & tomato juice
- Watercress and other salad leaves (but watch the dressing)
- Berries
- Grapefruit
- Melon
- Orange
- Pineapple

**Foods to watch**

- Pies & pastries
- Deep-fried food
- Cakes & biscuits
- Sponge & batter puddings
- Thick shakes
- Refined & processed foods
- Sweetened soft drinks
- Creamy liqueurs

## Ideas for Healthy Snacks

- Vegetable crudités with tomato salsa or tzatziki dip.
- Piece of fresh fruit or portion of fresh fruit salad (in unsweetened fruit juice).
- 3-4 Breadsticks.
- 2 water biscuits or oatcakes thinly spread with yeast extract or low-fat soft cheese.
- Handful of cherry tomatoes with 6 stoned olives.
- 5 Brazil nuts, dates or ready-to-eat dried apricots.
- Virgin Mary – tomato juice with Tabasco and Worcestershire sauce served with a stick of celery.
- Mug of vegetable (non-creamy) soup.
- 125 g pot of low-fat or natural bio yogurt
- Fruit ice lolly made with unsweetened fruit juice.

## Treats

You can occasionally indulge yourself with one of these tempting treats, but remember, they add unnecessary calories to your diet. Cut out such foods and drinks to lose weight faster or, step up your exercise routine, to help burn more calories.

- 1 standard glass (125 ml) of wine.
- half a pint lager / cider / beer / shandy.
- 1 spirit measure (25 ml) with diet mixer.
- 1 standard packet of crisps.
- 2 digestive biscuits.
- Slice of malt loaf, a toasted wholemeal hot cross bun with a lick of butter or a small piece of fruity flapjack.
- 1 fun-size chocolate bar.
- Small portion of dairy ice-cream.
- Fruit crudités (chunks of fresh fruit) with chocolate dip (melt just a couple of squares of dark chocolate and stir into reduced-fat Greek-style yogurt).

# Body contouring & toning exercises

## Warming-Up

Before you begin any workout routine, it's important to spend about 5 minutes or so doing some gentle warming-up exercises. This not only prepares the muscles and joints for the workout, thereby preventing any possible injury, but also increases the heart rate causing the blood to pump faster round the body. Consequently the harder the muscles work, the more beneficial the exercise will be.

## Basic warm-up movements

There are lots of warm-up exercises to choose from but basically they should be a blend of rhythmic stretching so that all parts of the body are limbered up and ready to go.

**SHOULDERS:** To loosen up tense shoulder and neck muscles, stand with your feet slightly apart, then roll the left shoulder backward ten times. Repeat with the right shoulder, at the same time shifting your weight from the left foot to the right foot.

**ARMS AND KNEES:** This is a great one for overall posture. Stand up straight, stomach tucked in, then swing both arms up and then swing them down, bending the knees as you bring the arms down in a gentle smooth action. Repeat 15 times.

**SIDE TO SIDE:** With your feet evenly spaced apart, knees gently bent and hands firmly on the hips, very slowly lean over to one side stretching the arm out at the same time as far as you can. Return to a standing position and stretch to the other side. Repeat four stretches on each side.

**WAISTING TIME:** This is good for the spine and waist. With your feet slightly parted, knees gently bent, hips facing forward, raise the arms nearly to shoulder level and, taking it easy, twist the body from side to side. Do four twists each side.

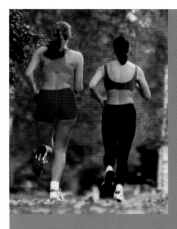

### TRAIN WITH A FRIEND

Teaming up with a 'fitness friend', someone who will workout with you and join you on walks and other sporting activities, is an excellent way to stay motivated. Having company and being able to support each other will reduce the temptation to miss any of your workout sessions and can also encourage you both to push yourselves a little harder.

# Trim & slim tips

Be prepared and follow some simple guidelines and dieting needn't be difficult or painful. Simply by making some small adjustments to your eating
habits and lifestyle, you'll be surprised how quickly you can drop that dress
size. Here are a few tips to help.

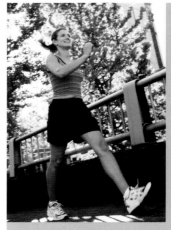

- Don't go food shopping when hungry or you'll risk being tempted by
  impulse buys that are probably not the healthiest choices.

- Stick to regular meal times, don't skip breakfast and try not to snack in
  between meals.

- Sit down to eat so you only associate eating with sitting at a table and
  avoid the habit of grazing on the hoof throughout the day.

- Eat slowly and chew your food thoroughly. It takes about 20 minutes
  for your brain to register a full stomach and by that time you can be
  over stuffed!

- Drink lots of water. A glass, when you're feeling hungry, will help to curb
  your appetite and make you feel full.

- Stick to low-fat cooking methods, such as boiling, steaming, grilling, stir-
  frying and microwaving.

- Restrict alcohol – it soon notches up a lot of empty calories.

- Eat a wide variety of foods so you don't get bored with your diet. The 7
  day diet plan includes many delicious ideas to get you started. You can
  then devise your own menus with other healthy recipes of your choice.

- Keep the fruit bowl full for weak moments. If you can't resist biscuits,
  crisps, chocolates and sweets, it's best not to buy them, thus keeping
  temptation out of sight.

- Always have healthy nibbles to hand (see *Healthy snacks and Free*
  *foods* on page 48) and plan meals ahead so you don't resort to less
  healthy or high calorie convenience meals or take-aways.

- We tend to snack when bored or if sitting watching TV, so keep busy.

- Sports activities are naturally
  good but also consider taking
  up new hobbies, such as a
  language class, so you have
  other interests to focus on.

- Treat yourself to a fabulous
  new outfit in the slimmer
  size you'd like to be. It will
  act as a powerful incentive
  and help to motivate you.

- Cut out a magazine picture
  of your ideal figure and stick
  it up on the fridge. This too
  will give you something
  positive to aim for.

# Body contouring & toning exercises

## The Workout

### BUTTOCK SQUEEZES

1. Lie on your back, knees bent, with your hands by your sides.

2. Keeping your abs tight, gently lift your hips off the floor and squeeze your bottom, then release.

3. Build up to 20 repetitions.

**Remember:**
• Keep your hips still.

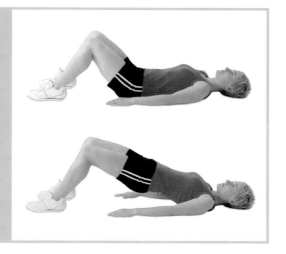

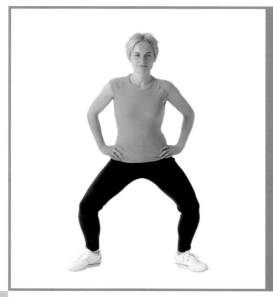

### SQUATS

1. Stand tall with your feet a little wider than shoulder-width apart, toes turned out slightly.

2. Place your hands on your hips.

3. Gently bend your knees in line with your toes, then slowly come up.

4. Do 8–12 repetitions.

**Remember:**
• Don't lock your knees when you come up.

# Recipes

## Strawberry Mousse

Silken tofu, widely available from larger supermarkets, gives this quick and easy mousse a lovely smooth texture. Other soft fruits, such as blackcurrants or mixed fruits of the forest can be used instead.

**SERVES 4**

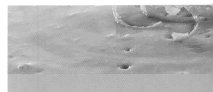

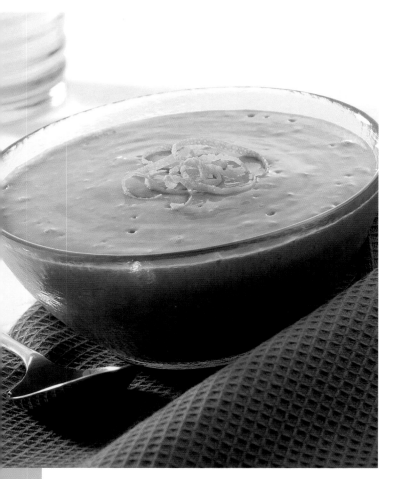

### INGREDIENTS

225 g (8 oz) silken tofu

450 g (1 lb) ripe strawberries, hulled

zest of 1 orange

1 tsp honey

### DIRECTIONS

1. Drain the tofu and place in a food processor or blender.

2. Roughly chop the strawberries and put in the food processor. Reserve some of the orange zest strips for decoration, and put the remaining zest in the food processor with the honey.

3. Process until smooth, spoon into dessert dishes and chill in the fridge.

4. Decorate with the reserved orange zest.

# Body contouring & toning exercises

## TUMMY TIGHTENER (THE PLANK)

1. Kneel on all fours, then go down on to your elbows.

2. Gently straighten your right leg to the back, your toes curled under, then straighten your left leg in the same way, so that both feet are together.

3. Pull your abs in tight and lower your hips.

4. Hold for 15 to 30 seconds, building up to 1 minute.

**Remember**
- Breathe.
- Keep your head in line with your body and your back flat.

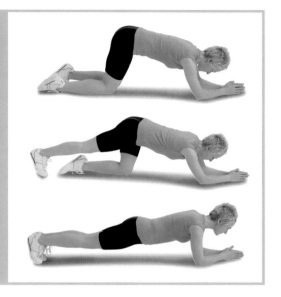

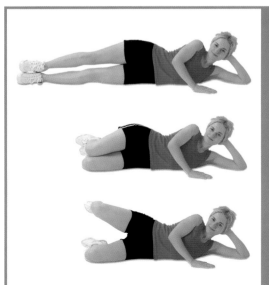

## OUTER THIGH RAISES

1. Lie on one side, hips facing forward, thighs together and your body in a straight line.

2. Support your head in one hand and place the other hand on the floor in front of you for support.

3. Bend both knees back.

4. Gently raise the top leg, then lower.

5. Do 6–7 repetitions, then repeat on the other side.

**Remember:**
- Squeeze your buttocks as you raise and lower your leg.
- Hips face forward.

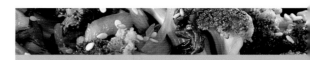

# Recipes

## Super Stir-fry

Fast and fresh, this stir-fry contains plentiful amounts of nourishing vegetables and seeds.

### SERVES 2

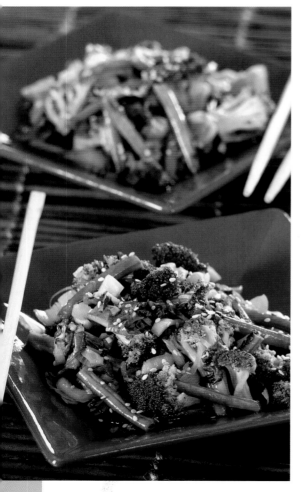

### INGREDIENTS

½ tbsp groundnut or vegetable oil

splash of toasted sesame oil

150 g (5½ oz) broccoli florets

2 spring onions, sliced

85 g (3 oz) pak choi, sliced

85 g (3 oz) fine green beans, trimmed

1 garlic clove, chopped

1 cm (½ in) piece of fresh ginger, peeled and
    finely chopped

1 tbsp apple juice

1 tbsp soy sauce

1 tbsp sesame seeds

### DIRECTIONS

1. Heat a frying pan or wok and add the groundnut and sesame oils. Add the broccoli, onion, pak choi and green beans. Stir-fry, tossing the vegetables continuously, for 6 minutes.

2. Add the garlic and ginger and stir-fry for another minute. Pour in the apple juice and soy sauce and cook for 1–2 minutes (add a little water if the stir-fry appears too dry) until the vegetables are just tender.

3. Sprinkle the sesame seeds on top and serve immediately.

# Body contouring & toning exercises

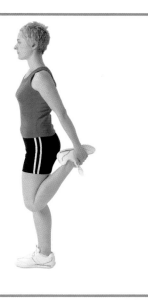

## THIGH STRETCHES

1. Stand tall with your feet hip-width apart, knees slightly bent.

2. Lift and bend one leg up behind you and hold the ankle with your hand.

3. Keep your knees aligned and the knee of the bent leg facing the floor, hips pushing slightly forward.

4. Hold, for 30 seconds then repeat on the other leg.

5. Feel the stretch at the front of the thigh.

**Note:**
You can use a wall or chair for support if you can't keep your balance in this position.

## LUNGES

1. Stand tall with your feet hip-width apart and your hands on your hips.

2. Take a big step forward, keeping your back heel raised and your weight on the ball of that foot.

3. Bend both knees as far as is comfortable, making sure the front knee does not go over the toe.

4. Hold for a count of one, then straighten both legs to return to the starting position.

5. Repeat on the other leg, alternating, until you have completed 8-12 repetitions on each leg.

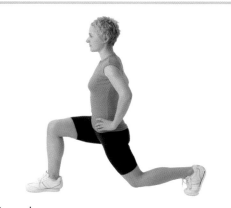

**Remember:**
- Keep your back straight at all times.
- Abs and buttock muscles are tight.
- Weight is evenly balanced between both legs.

# Recipes

## Saffron Chicken Rice

Brown rice, char-grilled chicken and fresh vegetables are combined here to make a simple, low-fat meal, providing useful amounts of fibre, vitamins and minerals. Serve with a green vegetable such as broccoli.

### SERVES 2

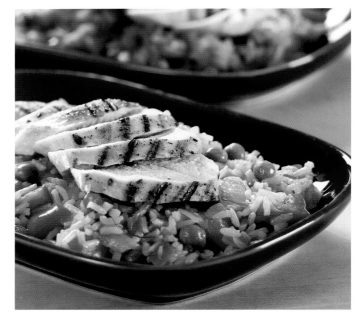

### INGREDIENTS

1 onion, diced

1½ tbsp olive oil, plus extra for griddling

1 red pepper, deseeded and diced

2 garlic cloves, chopped

2 tomatoes, deseeded and chopped

2 tsp tomato purée

large pinch of saffron

600 ml (1 pint) vegetable stock

175 g (6 oz) brown rice

2 skinless chicken breasts

55 g (2 oz) frozen peas

salt and freshly ground black pepper

### DIRECTIONS

1. Fry the onion in the oil for 8 minutes in a heavy-based sauté pan with a lid, until softened. Add the pepper, and garlic and sauté for a further 3 minutes over a medium heat.

2. Add the tomatoes and tomato purée to the pan, stir the saffron into the stock and pour in. Stir in the rice, bring to the boil, then reduce the heat. Cover, then simmer for 35 minutes or until the rice is tender. Stir occasionally and add extra stock or water, if required.

3. Meanwhile, brush the chicken breasts with a little oil. Heat a griddle pan and cook the chicken for 15–20 minutes, until cooked through.

4. Add the peas to the rice 3-4 minutes before the end of the cooking time. Season to taste. Place the rice in serving bowls and top with the chicken, cut into thin slices.

# Body contouring & toning exercises

### CURL-UPS

1. Lie on the floor with your feet hip-width apart and firmly on the floor, your knees bent.

2. Rest your hands on your thighs.

3. Using your tummy muscles, gently lift your shoulders off the floor, then lower.

4. Do 8–12 repetitions.

**Remember:**
- Breathe out when you come up, breathe in when you lower.
- Relax your head and neck and keep your chin off your chest.
- The movement should be fluid and continuous.
- Your back remains on the floor at all times.

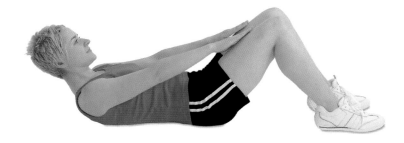

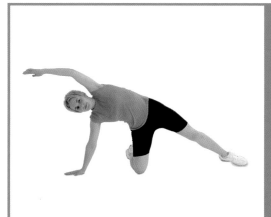

### SIDE STRETCHES

1. Kneel on your right knee, straighten your left leg to the side.

2. Place your right hand on the floor on the right side and gently bring your left arm over your head to stretch the side of the body.

3. Hold for a minimum of 10 seconds. Repeat on the other side.

**Remember:**
- Your right knee is directly under your right hip

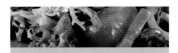

# Recipes

## Fresh Tuna Niçoise

A twist on the classic French salad made with fresh tuna steaks. Marinate for 30 minutes before cooking.

### SERVES 2

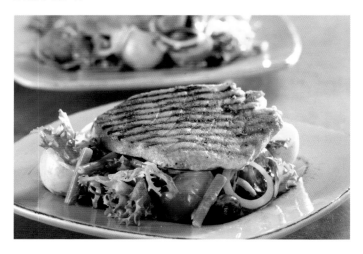

### INGREDIENTS

1 tbsp olive oil

1 tbsp fresh lemon juice

2 x 150 g (5¹/₂ oz) tuna steaks

250 g (9 oz) new potatoes,
  halved and cooked

85 g (3 oz) fine green beans,
  cooked

115 g (4 oz) mixed salad leaves

6 cherry tomatoes, halved

1 small red onion, sliced

handful black olives, stoned

salt and freshly ground black
  pepper

### DRESSING

1 tbsp extra virgin olive oil

¹/₂ tsp white wine vinegar

1 garlic clove, crushed

1 tbsp reduced-fat mayonnaise

### DIRECTIONS

1. Mix together the oil and lemon juice and season well. Place the tuna in a shallow dish and pour over the marinade. Chill for 30 minutes, turning the tuna occasionally.

2. Put the new potatoes, green beans, salad leaves, tomatoes, red onion and olives in a bowl.

3. Whisk together the ingredients for the dressing, then pour it over the salad and toss well.

4. Heat a griddle or frying pan until hot. Place the tuna steaks in the pan, brush with the marinade and cook for 3–5 minutes, turning once, until cooked on the outside and pink in the centre. Brush with the marinade while cooking.

5. Arrange the salad on serving plates and top each one with a tuna steak.

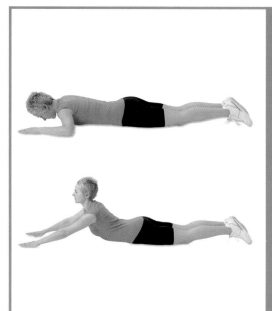

## ABDOMINAL STRETCH

1. Lie on your stomach, place your hands on the floor in front with your arms extended in front, your elbows slightly bent.

2. Gently push on your hands and lift your shoulders and head off the floor until you feel a stretch in your abdominal muscles.

3. Hold for a minimum of 10 seconds.

**Remember**

- Look straight ahead when you lift your head.
- Keep your hips and feet on the floor.
- Don't strain your back – only come up as far as is comfortable.

### TIP

Keep all the movements slow and controlled, remember to keep breathing easily and naturally and don't be too ambitious. You can gradually increase the number of repetitions you do for each exercise as you become stronger.

### KEEPING TRACK OF YOUR PROGRESS

Keeping an exercise diary can be a very helpful way of monitoring your progress. It's entirely up to you how you organise it. It could be totally factual with dates, durations and the type of exercises you performed, or you may choose to keep a record of your physical state and make notes on how you feel before, during and after your sessions.

# Recipes

## Mediterranean Sardines

Sardines are a great value buy both economically and nutritionally, providing beneficial omega-3 essential fatty acids. They are best marinated before cooking. Serve with crusty bread, grilled tomatoes and a green salad.

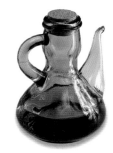

### SERVES 2

### INGREDIENTS

3 tbsp olive oil

$^{1}/_{2}$ lemon, zest and juice

1 garlic clove, crushed

1 tbsp chopped fresh oregano

1 tbsp snipped fresh chives

freshly ground black pepper

4–6 fresh sardines, depending
   on size, heads removed,
   gutted and cleaned

### DIRECTIONS

1. Mix together the olive oil, lemon zest, garlic, oregano, chives and pepper to season in a shallow dish large enough to hold the sardines in a single layer.

2. Arrange the sardines in the dish and turn them in the marinade. Leave for several hours or overnight in the fridge.

3. Preheat the grill to medium. Grill for about 10 minutes, turning them halfway through. The exact cooking time will depend on the size of the sardines: wait until they are golden and crispy on the outside. Squeeze the lemon juice over the fish before serving.

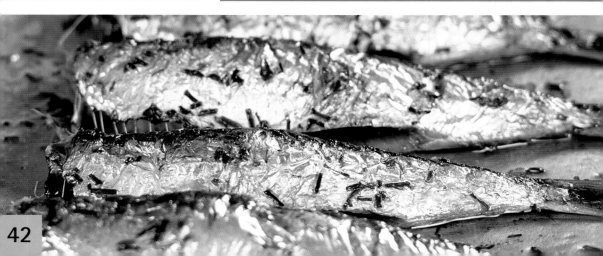

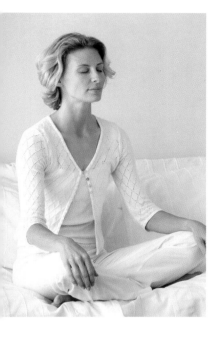

## Little time to exercise today?

Even if you haven't got much time to do a formal exercise session, here are some ideas for activities that might just give you some inspiration.

**Stand up and sit down:** When you are in the house alone or having a long phone call with a friend, try this exercise for a total lower body workout. Stand up and sit down repeatedly between sets of leg crossing. It works like a squat to tone the thighs and bottom.

**Deep breathing:** There is nothing quite so invigorating or relaxing as 5 minutes of deep, steady breathing to shake away those cobwebs. Deep breathing is also excellent for helping to de-stress. Try it when alone:
- If you are wearing a skirt or trousers, undo the waistband so there is space for you to relax your tummy.
- Close your eyes, slowly breathe in, holding that breath to the count of 5, and to the count of five slowly exhale through your mouth.
- Repeat again several times.

### Cooling down

Just as you need to prepare the body for exercising with warming-up exercises, you also need to cool it down after you have finished. After all, your body has been through quite an ordeal! You will find lots of different warming-up and cooling-down exercises in various books but here are a few favourites for you to try.

**SPINE RELAXER:** Sitting cross-legged, stomach held in, bend forward and hold your arms out on the floor in front of you. Hold for the count of 10 and then relax.

**BACK AND ARMS:** This may sound rather tricky but it is very relaxing. Again sitting cross-legged on the floor with your back straight, clench your hands behind your back, clasp your fingers together and gently pull on them for a count of 10. Then relax.

**AB TENSER:** Lie face down on the floor, with your elbows slightly bent so that they are under your shoulders. Making sure the forearms and elbows remain on the floor, raise both head and shoulders very slowly. Hold this position for a count of 6, then relax.

# Recipes

## Guacamole with Roasted Vegetables

A colourful selection of roasted vegetables, cooked with fresh rosemary, and served with a creamy avacado dip.

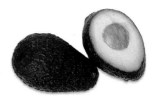

**SERVES 2**

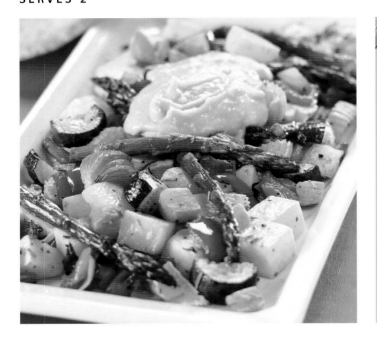

### INGREDIENTS

selection of vegetables
(Choose from butternut
  squash, red pepper,
  asparagus, red onion,
  courgettes, carrots and
  fennel), cut into chunks
1 tbsp olive oil
few sprigs fresh rosemary
1 avocado, stone removed
1 small garlic clove, crushed
1 tbsp fresh lemon juice

### DIRECTIONS

1. Preheat the oven to 200°C/400°F/Gas Mark 6. Place your chosen selection of vegetables in a roasting dish. Toss the vegetables in the olive oil using your hands. Place the sprigs of rosemary in between and roast in the oven for 30–40 minutes until the vegetables are tender and golden.

2. Meanwhile, make the guacamole. Scoop out the avocado flesh using a spoon. Mash with the garlic and lemon juice until fairly smooth and creamy.

3. To serve, remove the rosemary sprigs and arrange the roasted vegetables on a plate. Top with a spoonful of guacamole. Serve with wholemeal pitta bread.

# Spot reducing for problem areas

As well as slimming down and firming up your whole body, there may well be particular areas that you need to work on. Whether it's a flabby stomach, saggy bottom, spreading hips or an undefined waist that you're unhappy with, add these specific exercises to your workout routine to improve your shape, curves and vital statistics. If you have one particular area that you feel needs more work than another, then simply spend more time working on that. You'll notice the difference after just 2-3 weeks.

## Tummy & waist exercises

### TUMMY TIGHTENER

1. Kneel down on all fours, with your hands directly under your shoulders, your elbows slightly bent, your knees directly under your hips.

2. Look down at the floor, keeping your head in line with the rest of the body.

3. Relax your abs completely, then slowly pull them up and in tight.

4. Hold for 30 seconds, building up to 1 minute, then relax.

**Remember:**
- Keep your spine still and flat.
- Don't lock your elbows.

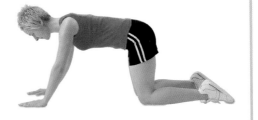

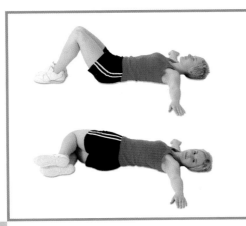

### WAIST STRETCH

1. Lie on your back with your knees bent and your arms at shoulder level.

2. Gently drop both knees to one side and turn your head in the opposite direction.

3. Hold, then slowly repeat on the other side.

**Remember:**
- Keep your feet and both shoulders on the floor.
- Breathe easily throughout.

# Recipes

## Wild Rice Salad with Cucumber & Orange

### SERVES 4

#### DIRECTIONS

1. Cook the rice in a large pan of lightly salted boiling water for 15-18 minutes or according to the pack instructions, until the rice is tender.

2. To make the dressing, put the garlic, vinegar, olive oil and seasoning into a screw-top jar and shake vigorously.

3. Drain the rice and turn into a large bowl. Pour over the dressing and mix in. Add the peppers, cucumber, orange, tomatoes, onion and parsley and toss together.

### INGREDIENTS

225 g (8 oz) basmati and wild rice

1 garlic clove, crushed

1 tbsp balsamic vinegar

2 tbsp olive oil

sea salt and freshly ground black pepper

1 each of red, yellow and orange peppers, deseeded and diced

1/2 cucumber, diced

1 orange, peeled, pith removed and chopped

3 ripe tomatoes, chopped

1 red onion, finely chopped

generous handful chopped flat-leaf parsley

## Fennel & orange salad

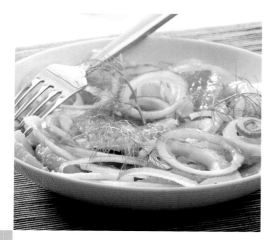

### SERVES 4

### INGREDIENTS

3 oranges, peeled and sliced, flesh of 2 and juice of 1

1 bulb Florence fennel, thinly sliced

1 red onion, peeled and sliced into thin rings

2 tbsp balsamic vinegar

### DIRECTIONS

1 Arrange the orange slices in a shallow dish then layer the fennel and onion on top.

2 Mix the orange juice with the vinegar and drizzle over the salad.

## WALKING LEGS (SCISSORS)

1. Lie on your back with your arms by your sides, legs extended straight up.

2. Contract your abdominals and 'walk' in the air with your legs, taking one leg up towards your head and the other down towards the ground.

3. Make the movements quite small to begin with then, as you build up strength, start to take the legs lower.

**Remember:**

- Keep the abdominal contraction as you move – if you start to lose it, you've gone too far.

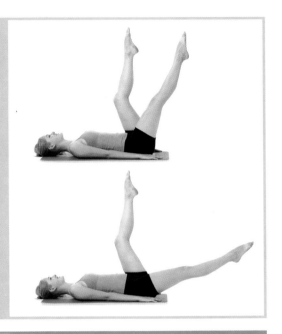

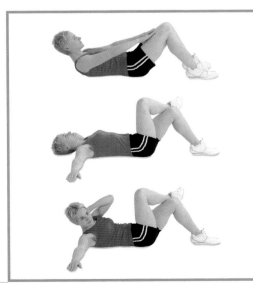

## WAIST TIGHTENER

1. Lie on the floor with your feet hip-width apart and firmly on the floor, with your knees bent.

2. Place your left hand behind your head, with your elbow bent. Place your right foot on your left knee.

3. Place your other hand on the floor for support.

4. Tighten your abs and slowly curl up and over diagonally, bringing your shoulder round to meet your knee, then lower.

5. Do 8–12 repetitions, then repeat on the other side.

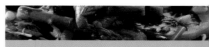

## Asparagus & Tomato Salad

Although you can buy imported asparagus throughout the year, you can't beat home-grown for quality and flavour during early summer. Here it's added to a tomato salad for a luxurious starter.

### SERVES 4

### DIRECTIONS

1. Steam the asparagus spears for about 8 minutes or until tender. Rinse under cold running water to prevent them cooking any further, then cut into 5 cm (2 in) pieces.

2. Arrange the salad leaves on 4 plates to form the base of the salad. Place the sliced tomatoes in a circle on top and the asparagus in the centre.

3. Sprinkle the black olives and pine nuts over the top. Put the lemon juice olive oil, mustard and vinegar in a screw-top jar and season to taste with black pepper. Shake vigorously and drizzle over the salad.

### INGREDIENTS

225 g (8 oz) asparagus spears

45g (1 1/2 oz) lamb's lettuce

100g (3 1/2 oz) rocket or mizuna leaves

450 g (1 lb) ripe tomatoes, sliced

12 black olives, stoned and chopped

1 tbsp pine nuts, toasted

1 tsp lemon juice

1 tbsp olive oil

1 tsp wholegrain mustard

2 tbsp balsamic vinegar

freshly ground black pepper

### RECIPE TIP

Always cook asparagus quickly and be careful not to overcook it. Steaming is the best method for protecting the delicate tips. Thicker spears will take slightly longer to cook than thin spears. If the stems seem coarse, trim off the woody ends before cooking.

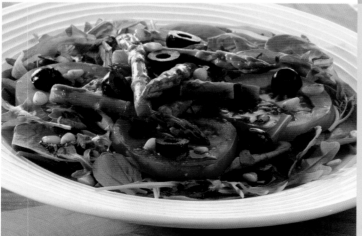

## AB CRUNCHERS

1. Lie on your back with your knees bent and your feet flat on the floor, hip-width apart.

2. Tilt your pelvis until your lower back is pressed flat against the floor.

3. Rest your hands lightly against the side of your head.

4. Now slowly lift your head and shoulders a little way off the floor.

5. Hold for a few seconds and then lower back down to the floor.

6. Repeat 15–20 times.

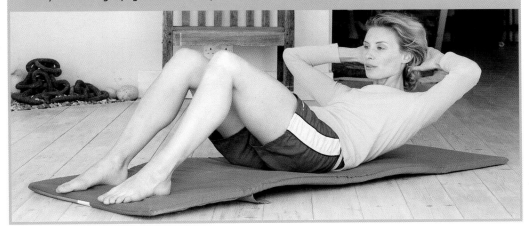

**Note:** The plank, curl-ups and side stretches included in the whole body workout, are also particularly good toning exercises for the waist and tummy.

## Bottom exercises

### GLUTE SQUEEZES

Sit in a chair with your back straight. Contract your abdominals and squeeze your buttocks, holding for 3–5 counts, then release for 2. Repeat the sequence 10 times, gradually building to 20.

Tip:
You can practise the glute squeeze at any time, wherever you are. For fast results and firmer buttocks, repeat the sequence 4–5 times throughout the day.

# Recipes

## Luxury Muesli

This skin-nourishing muesli makes a perfect start to the day served with live natural bio yogurt and topped with sliced strawberries.

**SERVES 6**

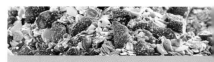

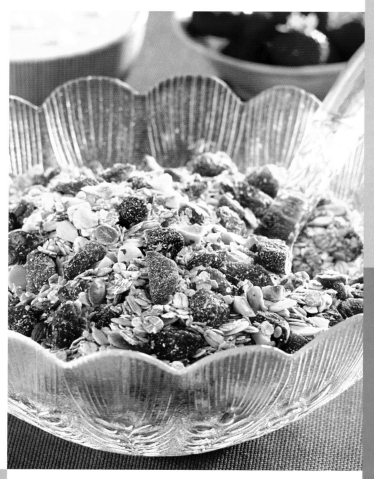

### INGREDIENTS

50 g (2 oz) sunflower seeds

25 g (1 oz) pumpkin seeds

25 g (1 oz) sesame seeds

115 g (4 oz) porridge oats

115 g (4 oz) barley flakes

115 g (4 oz) wheat flakes

115 g (4 oz) raisins

115 g (4 oz) roasted whole hazelnuts, chopped

85 g (3 oz) almonds, roughly chopped

115 g (4 oz) dried apricots, roughly chopped

50 g (2 oz) dried cherries.

### DIRECTIONS

**1** Lightly toast the sunflower, pumpkin and sesame seeds in a dry frying pan until just golden, tossing them regularly to prevent burning. Leave to cool.

**2** Mix the toasted seeds with the rest of the ingredients. Store in an airtight container

## KNEELING BUTTOCK TIGHTENER

1. Kneel on all fours in a box position with your hands on the floor.

2. Gently go down on to your elbows, extend one leg to the back and bend at the knee so that it's in line with your hips and the heel is facing the ceiling. Your back is flat (this is the starting position).

3. Squeezing your buttock muscles, gently raise your leg, then lower to the starting position.

4. Do 8–12 repetitions, then repeat on the other leg.

**Remember:**
• Don't move your hips.
• Keep your heel facing the ceiling.
• Make sure your back is flat.

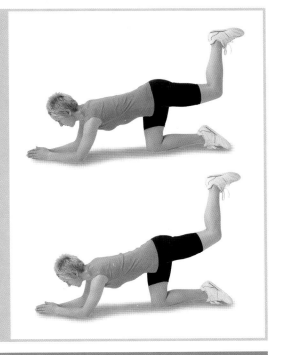

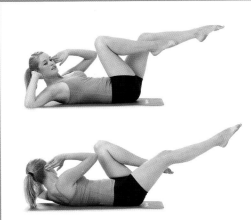

## CYCLING

1. Lie on your back with your legs raised and your knees slightly bent, hands resting lightly behind your ears.

2. Contract your abdominals and twist your body from side to side, bringing each knee towards your chest in a 'pedalling' motion and touching that same knee with the opposite elbow as you do so.

3. Start with 10 repetitions for each side, gradually increasing to 20. Repeat the sequence on alternate days.

# 7 day diet plan

| | BREAKFAST. | LUNCH | DINNER |
|---|---|---|---|
| **DAY 5** | Canned prunes (or dried fruit compote) in fruit juice Luxury Muesli (see page 38) or sugar-free supermarket muesli with semi-skimmed milk. | Greek salad (made with cubes of feta cheese, chopped tomatoes, cucumber, red onions, olives and mixed salad leaves drizzled with a little vinaigrette dressing). 2 sesame seed grissini | Saffron Chicken Rice (see page 44). Exotic fruit salad (sliced oranges, kiwi fruit, lychees and black grapes in unsweetened apple juice with some chopped stem ginger added). |
| **DAY 6** | Unsweetened fruit juice (Orange, grapefruit, cranberry and tomato juices are all a good source of vitamin C. Go for a pure fruit juice rather than a juice drink, or squeeze your own fresh fruit). Boiled egg with wholemeal toast (lightly spread with low-fat spread and yeast extract) | Mediterranean Sardines (see page 42) served with crusty bread, grilled tomatoes and a green salad. Alternatively, serve with Wild Rice Salad with Cucumber and Orange (see page 40) of Fennel and Orange Salad (see page 40). For speed, buy ready cleaned and scaled sardines. | Meatballs with tomato sauce and spaghetti (pan-fry bought chilled meatballs in a non-stick pan then pour over a good quality tomato sauce for pasta and heat through. Serve with wholewheat spaghetti. If liked, sprinkle with a little freshly grated Parmesan) Peach Melba (small scoop of vanilla dairy ice-cream served with sliced peaches and drizzled with fresh raspberry sauce – blend raspberries in a blender or processor with a squeeze of lemon juice and a little icing sugar to taste) |
| **DAY 7** | Greek-style yogurt (reduced-fat) topped with sliced banana and scattered with fresh blueberries Wholemeal muffin, toasted and spread with peanut butter | Asparagus and Tomato Salad (see page 39) Grilled steak with boiled new potatoes Strawberry Mousse (see page 46) | Vegetable Soup (such as carrot and coriander or lentil). It can be any flavour you choose and quite hearty but not rich and creamy. Multi-grain bap (unbuttered) |

# Spot reducing for problem areas

## SITTING BUTTOCK STRETCH

1. Sit in a cross-legged position (right leg under, left leg over), with your hands on the floor in front of you.

2. Slowly start walking forward with your hands until you feel a stretch in your left buttock.

3. Hold, then switch legs over and repeat so you feel the stretch in the right buttock.

**Remember:**
• Ease forward from the hip.

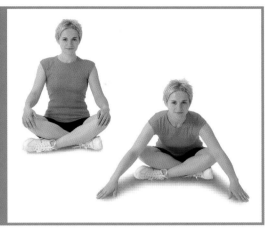

**Note:** Squats and lunges included in the whole body workout, are also particularly good toning exercises for the bottom.

## Hip and thigh exercises

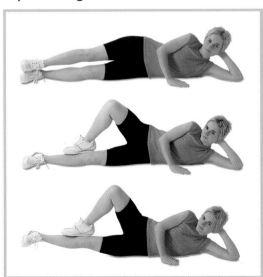

### INNER THIGH RAISES

1. Lie on your side, hips facing forward, thighs together and your body in a straight line.

2. Gently come up on to your elbow for support.

3. Now bend your top leg and place your foot on the inner part of the bottom leg.

4. Raise the lower leg off the floor, then lower.

5. Do 8–12 repetitions, then repeat on the other leg.

**Remember:**
• Hips face forward.
• Body remains aligned.

# 7 day diet plan

| | BREAKFAST | LUNCH | DINNER |
|---|---|---|---|
| DAY 1 | Glass of unsweetened fruit juice. Luxury Muesli (see page 38) or sugar-free supermarket muesli with semi-skimmed milk. | Chicken salad sandwich ( thick sliced wholemeal bread lightly spread with low-fat spread or reduced fat mayonnaise and filled with lean chicken breast and plenty of salad). 1 crisp apple or juicy pear | Guacamole with Roasted Vegetables (see page 41) 1 wholemeal pitta bread (toasted and cut into fingers) Fresh raspberries with spoonful of reduced-fat Greek-style yogurt or low-fat crème fraîche. |
| DAY 2 | Unsweetened grapefruit segments 2 slices of wholemeal toast thinly spread with low-fat spread and marmite, reduced-sugar marmalade or jam or peanut butter. | Ham and pineapple pasta salad (wholewheat pasta shapes tossed with diced, lean, cooked ham, canned pineapple cubes in natural juice and chopped spring onions with reduced-fat mayonnaise. Scatter with some chopped walnuts) 1 live bio fruit yogurt | Fresh Tuna Nicoise ( see page 43) Large slice of fresh, juicy melon |
| DAY 3 | Glass of unsweetened fruit juice Porridge (made with semi-skimmed milk) sweetened with a little sugar / honey | Jacket potato (no butter) topped with baked beans (preferably with reduced sugar) or cottage cheese with prawns or a little grated mature Cheddar with chutney 1 peach | Grilled pork steak with Super stir-fry (see page 45) Poached pear (cooked in unsweetened apple juice) drizzled with dark chocolate sauce |
| DAY 4 | Mango and strawberry smoothie (blend 1 fresh peeled and stoned mango with 100 g / 3½ oz fresh strawberries. Dilute with a little orange juice if too thick). Poached egg on wholemeal toast | Slice of Vegetable pizza (go for one with a thick layer of tomato and not too much cheese) Mixed side salad (avoid creamy dressings. Choose a low-fat dressing or use a little vinaigrette) | Sloppy Joes (bolognese sauce made with lean minced beef, mushrooms and peppers served on a toasted bap). |

# Spot reducing for problem areas

## HIP FLEXOR STRETCH

1. Kneel on your left leg, keeping the right leg bent, with your right foot firmly on the floor.

2. Place your hands on either side of your right foot for support.

3. Gently raise the left knee off the floor and straighten the left leg.

4. Lower your hips towards the floor.

5. Hold, then repeat on the other side.

**Remember:**
• Don't bounce.
• Don't lock your knee.

**Note:**
If you can't keep your back leg straight, keep your knee on the floor.

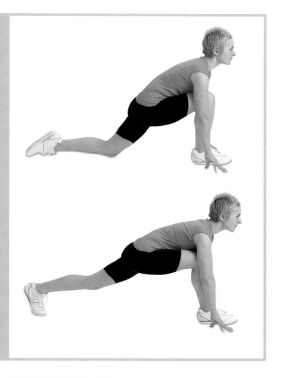

## PILLOW SQUEEZES

Lie on your back with your knees bent, feet together, hands by your sides. Place a pillow between your knees, contract the abdominals and exhale, squeezing the inner thighs together for a count of 10 as you do so. Release. Repeat 10 times.

## FOOT ROTATIONS

Position yourself following steps 1 & 2 of the Inner thigh raise exercise, but with your lower leg bent comfortably behind. Now raise your top leg as far as you can and rotate the ankle and foot clockwise. Slowly lower and repeat the leg raise and rotation 10 times. Turn over and repeat on the other side.

**Note:** Outer thigh raises and thigh stretches included in the whole body workout, are also particularly good toning exercises for the hips and thighs.

# Choose a healthy diet

Achieving a fit and toned body requires eating healthily as much as taking regular exercise and leading an active lifestyle. Food is needed as fuel for the body but it's not just a matter of eating to satisfy your appetite and meeting your energy needs. The choices you make and nutrient quality of your food greatly influence how you look and feel.

Use this sample weekly diet plan as a blueprint for a healthy diet. It's designed to be used as a guide so you get into the swing of making healthy and varied food choices and eating regular meals that are satisfying and enjoyable. You don't need to do any tedious calorie counting, because by making sensible choices and cooking by low-fat cooking methods, your appetite will naturally control how much you eat. You can mix and match the menu ideas to suit your lifestyle but do include all the fruits and vegetables (although they can be swapped for alternative choices) to make sure you are eating your '5 a day'. After week 1, you can then design your own menus following these guidelines:

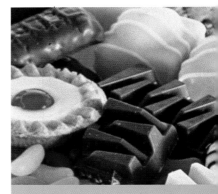

- Eat 3 meals a day - breakfast, lunch and dinner. Don't skip meals and in particular, make time for breakfast to get your day off to a healthy start.
- Eat a wide variety of different foods. This will help ensure your diet includes all the nutrients needed for good health.
- Go for lean meat, fish and poultry, starchy carbohydrates like bread, rice, pasta and potatoes and aim for at least 5 portions of fruit and vegetables daily. Wholegrain cereals, like wholemeal bread, brown rice and oats are particularly satisfying to eat and like fruit, vegetables and pulses are good sources of fibre, needed for a healthy digestion.
- Cut down on high fat and sugary foods and unnecessary snacks between meals. For weak moments, choose a low-fat snack, such as a piece of fruit or some raw vegetable crudités with a tomato salsa or tzatziki dip.
- You can have up to 300 ml /¹/₂ pint semi-skimmed milk each day for hot drinks or try herbal teas, hot lemon, blackcurrant or Bovril as alternatives.
- Drink plenty of water – aim for 6 - 8 glasses daily. Add ice and a slice of lemon or if you're not keen on plain water, add a splash of fruit juice or cordial to sparkling mineral water.

## TREATS

Cakes, biscuits, crisps, sweets and chocolates, rich puddings and alcoholic drinks are not essential in terms of providing nutrients in a healthy diet so try and restrict them to a minimum. There's no need to ban them completely but think of them as occasional treats. Remember it's these types of foods that can so easily bump up your calorie intake and if you consume more calories than you use, the excess will be stored as fat.

# Spot reducing for problem areas

## Arm and chest exercises

### UPPER ARMS

1. Fill a 2 litre empty plastic pop bottle with water to use as a weight.

2. Sit on a seat.

3. Take the bottle in one hand and move it over your head, palm facing inward.

4. Slowly bend your elbow so that you are bringing the bottle down to your shoulder but without altering the upper arm position.

5. Lift the arm up and repeat the same process again.

6. Do this exercise 6 times with one arm and 6 with the other.

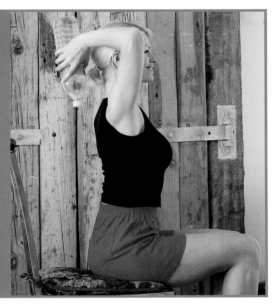

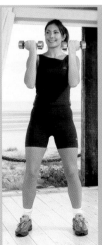

### BICEP CURLS

1. Stand with both feet hip-width apart and arms down by your sides, holding a light weight (such as a can of beans) in each hand.

2. Bring the arms slightly forward, raise the hands, then bend and lift the elbows up and back, pushing hard.

3. Lower the arms back down and repeat 20 times.

### ARM CIRCLES

1. Stand with your feet hip-width apart. Raise your right arm up in front of you then curve it up and over your head and back down and round in a big circle.

2. Repeat for 5–10 circles then reverse the direction. Repeat for the other side. Now circle both arms at the same time, first in one direction, then the other, 5 more times.

3. Keep your shoulders relaxed throughout this move. You will need to make the circles much smaller when you work both arms together. Concentrate on making the circling movement as smooth and even as possible.

## Exercise those muscles

Good posture won't come about just by willing yourself to stand straight and tall. You need to build up muscle power to hold you up in the correct posture so that you can stand properly without having to consciously think about it. The main muscles that influence posture are the buttocks, the hip flexors and the abdominals. A regular workout doing the body contouring and toning exercises, particularly the exercises working on these muscles, will noticeably help to improve your posture.

### HIP FLEXORS

The hip flexors are a group of muscles that run from the hip to the lower spine or at various points along the thigh bone. They work in opposition to the buttocks, helping you move your hips, raise your thighs and bring your knees up towards your body as you walk.

If you do a lot of sitting and no exercise, your hip flexors are likely to be tight, while at the same time your buttocks are probably slack and lack tone. The tighter your hip flexors get, the more they pull on the muscles in your buttocks, stretching them and making them even slacker. This is a good example of how a weakness in one part of your body has a knock-on effect, causing a problem in another part of your body. Ideally, both the buttocks and hip flexors would be equally toned and flexible and would therefore exert a balanced pressure on each other. When they get unbalanced, postural problems and sometimes injury result.

### ABDOMINAL MUSCLES

The muscles in your abdomen stabilise your lower back and hold your body in alignment. Poor muscle tone in the abdomen is usually caused by carrying too much weight or exercising too little. Women who have just had a baby will have poor abdominal muscle tone because their muscles have been stretched during pregnancy.

Poor muscle tone can be corrected with exercise. Sit-ups or curl-ups can be useful but they must be done properly so that the abdominal muscles really are doing the work.

### BUTTOCK MUSCLES

The buttocks stabilise the hips, hold the pelvis in the right position and balance the entire hip area. In order to do all that work, they need to be both toned and flexible. Even just getting up and walking for 20-30 minutes a day will improve the muscle tone of your buttocks. Climbing stairs is also helpful.

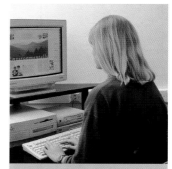

**Be sure to work at the right height so as to sit up straight and not strain your neck. Get up and stretch regularly.**

# Your weekly exercise routine

This is designed just as an example of how much exercise you should plan to include in your daily lifestyle. You can vary it to suit your own schedule, including your own favourite activities and specific exercises that work on particular areas. The key points are that it is varied and regular. As the weeks progress, and your strength and stamina improves, you can increase the timings or number of repetitions for particular exercises. Keep it up and it won't be long before you are rewarded with that curvy shape and your target size.

| | A.M. | MID-DAY | P.M. |
|---|---|---|---|
| DAY 1 | 5 minutes skipping | 20 minute brisk walk | 10-15 minute workout (remember to include warm-up exercises) |
| DAY 2 | 10–15 minutes on spot reducing exercises | 15 minute swim | 20 - 30 minute bike ride |
| DAY 3 | 15 minute workout | 20 minute brisk walk | game of badminton (or other sport) |
| DAY 4 | early-bird swim | 20 minute brisk walk | 20 minute workout including chosen spot reducing exercises |
| DAY 5 | 5 minutes skipping | 20 minute brisk walk | Dance class |
| DAY 6 | circuit training class or 30 minute workout including spot reducing exercises | 30 minutes gardening | 20 minute brisk walk |
| DAY 7 | 20 –30 minute workout including chosen spot reducing exercises | Rest | 1 hour bike ride or brisk walk |

# The importance of good posture

Good posture is the cornerstone of a fit body and a good appearance. When you are standing straight, you will look and feel more poised and confident, your back will be under far less strain and your clothes will hang better.

## Good posture

The correct way to stand is with your head up and centred over your shoulders, your shoulders back and your back flat with a slight hollow in the small of the back. Your hips should be straight, not tilted forward, back, or to either side. You can visualise correct posture by imagining that you are a puppet with a string coming out of the top of your head. As the string pulls up, your whole body comes into alignment, one part stacked comfortably over the other. Good posture looks natural and relaxed, neither rigid nor slouched. It also keeps your muscles balanced and toned in relation to one another.

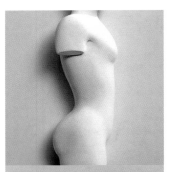

In its correct posture, the back is flat with a slight hollow, and the shoulders are back with the head centred over them.

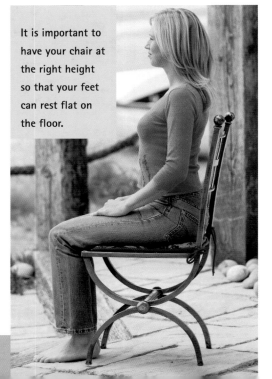

It is important to have your chair at the right height so that your feet can rest flat on the floor.

## Are you sitting comfortably?

A lot of us spend our working lives sitting at a desk. The way that we sit can make a big difference to our posture and our health because sitting puts much more strain on the lower back than standing, which is five times more stressful than lying down.

You should sit up straight with your feet flat on the floor, your knees slightly higher than your hips, and your lower back supported. The desk should be at the right height so that you can fit your chair and your knees beneath it. If you work at a computer, the screen and any paperwork should be at eye level so that you don't need to strain your neck by looking up or down. Your arms should be at right angles to your keyboard. Move the seat of your chair and your back rest up and down until you can achieve the correct position. Once you are sitting comfortably, remember to get up and stretch once in a while.